Outcomes Research in Surgical Oncology

Guest Editor

CLIFFORD Y. KO, MD, MS, MSHS

SURGICAL ONCOLOGY CLINICS OF NORTH AMERICA

www.surgonc.theclinics.com

Consulting Editor
NICHOLAS J. PETRELLI, MD

July 2012 • Volume 21 • Number 3

SAUNDERS an imprint of ELSEVIER, Inc.

W.B. SAUNDERS COMPANY

A Division of Elsevier Inc.

1600 John F. Kennedy Boulevard • Suite 1800 • Philadelphia, PA 19103-2899

http://www.theclinics.com

SURGICAL ONCOLOGY CLINICS OF NORTH AMERICA Volume 21, Number 3
July 2012 ISSN 1055-3207, ISBN-13: 978-1-4557-4949-2

Editor: Jessica McCool

Surgical Oncology Clinics of North America (ISSN 1055-3207) is published quarterly by Elsevier Inc., 360 Park Avenue South, New York, NY 10010-1710. Months of publication are January, April, July, and October. Business and Editorial Offices: 1600 John F. Kennedy Blvd., Ste. 1800, Philadelphia, PA 19103-2899. Customer Service Office: 3251 Riverport Lane, Maryland Heights, MO 63043. Periodicals postage paid at New York, NY and additional mailing offices. Subscription prices are $263.00 per year (US individuals), $386.00 (US institutions) $130.00 (US student/resident), $302.00 (Canadian individuals), $480.00 (Canadian institutions), $186.00 (Canadian student/resident), $377.00 (foreign individuals), $480.00 (foreign institutions), and $186.00 (foreign student/resident). Foreign air speed delivery is included in all *Clinics* subscription prices. All prices are subject to change without notice. **POSTMASTER**: Send address changes to *Surgical Oncology Clinics of North America*, Elsevier Health Science Division, Subscription Customer Service, 3251 Riverport Lane, Maryland Heights, MO 63043. **Customer Service: 1-800-654-2452 (US and Canada). 314-447-8871 (outside U.S. and Canada). Fax: 314-447-8029. E-mail: journalscustomerservice-usa@elsevier.com** (for print support); **journalsonline support-usa@elsevier.com** (for online support).

Reprints. For copies of 100 or more, of articles in this publication, please contact the Commercial Reprints Department, Elsevier Inc., 360 Park Avenue South, New York, New York 10010-1710. Tel. 212-633-3813; Fax: 212-462-1935; E-mail: reprints@elsevier.com.

Surgical Oncology Clinics of North America is covered in *MEDLINE/PubMed (Index Medicus)* and *EMBASE/ Excerpta Medica, Current Contents/Clinical Medicine,* and *ISI/BIOMED.*

Printed and bound by CPI Group (UK) Ltd, Croydon, CR0 4YY
Transferred to Digital Print 2012

Contributors

CONSULTING EDITOR

NICHOLAS J. PETRELLI, MD
Bank of America Endowed Medical Director, Helen F. Graham Cancer Center at Christiana
Care Health System, Newark, Delaware

GUEST EDITOR

CLIFFORD Y. KO, MD, MS, MSHS
Department of Surgery, University of California, Los Angeles, Los Angeles, California;
Division of Research and Optimal Patient Care, American College of Surgeons,
Chicago, Illinois

AUTHORS

DAVID J. BENTREM, MD, MS
Division of Surgical Oncology, Department of Surgery, Northwestern University Feinberg
School of Medicine, Chicago, Illinois

KARL Y. BILIMORIA, MD, MS
Division of Surgical Oncology, Department of Surgery, Institute for Healthcare Studies,
Surgical Outcomes and Quality Improvement Center, Northwestern University Feinberg
School of Medicine, Chicago, Illinois

JANICE N. CORMIER, MD, MPH
Associate Professor, Department of Surgical Oncology, The University of Texas MD
Anderson Cancer Center, Houston, Texas

KATE D. CROMWELL, MS
Research Data Coordinator, Department of Surgical Oncology, The University of Texas
MD Anderson Cancer Center, Houston, Texas

JUSTIN B. DIMICK, MD, MPH
Assistant Professor of Surgery, Center for Healthcare Outcomes and Policy (CHOP),
University of Michigan, Ann Arbor, Michigan

NESTOR F. ESNAOLA, MD, MPH, MBA
Associate Professor, Division of Surgical Oncology, Department of Surgery, Medical
University of South Carolina, Charleston, South Carolina

MARVELLA E. FORD, PhD
Associate Professor, Division of Biostatistics and Epidemiology, Department of Medicine,
Medical University of South Carolina, Charleston, South Carolina

AMIR A. GHAFERI, MD, MS
Chief Resident in Surgery, Center for Healthcare Outcomes and Policy (CHOP), University of Michigan, Ann Arbor, Michigan

MELINDA MAGGARD GIBBONS, MD, MSHS
Department of Surgery, University of California, Los Angeles, Los Angeles, California

CAPRICE C. GREENBERG, MD, MPH
Wisconsin Surgical Outcomes Research Program, Department of Surgery, University of Wisconsin Hospitals and Clinics, Madison, Wisconsin

PATRICK GRUSENMEYER, FACHE, ScD
Senior Vice President, Cancer and Imaging Services, Helen F. Graham Cancer Center at Christiana Care Health System, Newark, Delaware

YUE-YUNG HU, MD, MPH
Department of Surgery, Center for Surgery and Public Health, Brigham and Women's Hospital; Department of Surgery, Beth Israel Deaconess Medical Center, Boston, Massachusetts

BRANDON K. ISARIYAWONGSE, MD
Resident, Department of Urology, Glickman Urological and Kidney Institute, Cleveland Clinic Foundation, Cleveland, Ohio

MICHAEL W. KATTAN, PhD
Chairman, Department of Quantitative and Health Sciences, Cleveland Clinic Foundation, Cleveland, Ohio

CLIFFORD Y. KO, MD, MS, MSHS
Department of Surgery, University of California, Los Angeles, Los Angeles, California; Division of Research and Optimal Patient Care, American College of Surgeons, Chicago, Illinois

ELISE H. LAWSON, MD, MSHS
Department of Surgery, University of California, Los Angeles, Los Angeles, California

KELLIE L. MATHIS, MD
Department of Surgery, Division of Colon and Rectal Surgery, Mayo Clinic, Rochester, Minnesota

RYAN P. MERKOW, MD
Department of Surgery and Surgical Outcomes and Quality Improvement Center, Northwestern University Feinberg School of Medicine; Division of Research and Optimal Patient Care, American College of Surgeons, Chicago, Illinois; Department of Surgery, University of Colorado School of Medicine, Aurora, Colorado

HEIDI NELSON, MD
Department of Surgery, Division of Colon and Rectal Surgery, Mayo Clinic, Rochester, Minnesota

NICHOLAS J. PETRELLI, MD
Bank of America Endowed Medical Director, Helen F. Graham Cancer Center at Christiana Care Health System, Newark, Delaware

RAPHAEL E. POLLOCK, MD
Professor and Head for the Division of Surgery, Department of Surgical Oncology,
The University of Texas MD Anderson Cancer Center, Houston, Texas

MATTHEW M. ROCHEFORT, MD
Research Fellow, Department of Surgery, David Geffen School of Medicine at UCLA,
Los Angeles, California

ANDREW K. STEWART, MA
Manager, National Cancer Data Base, Cancer Programs, American College of Surgeons,
Chicago, Illinois

JAMES S. TOMLINSON, MD, PhD
Associate Professor of Surgery, Department of Surgery, University of California,
Los Angeles, David Geffen School of Medicine at UCLA; Chief, Surgical Oncology,
Greater Los Angeles VA Medical Center, Los Angeles, California

RICHELLE T. WILLIAMS, MD
Research Fellow, Department of Surgery, University of Chicago Medical Center; Cancer
Programs, American College of Surgeons, Chicago, Illinois

DAVID P. WINCHESTER, MD
Medical Director, Cancer Programs, American College of Surgeons, Chicago;
Department of Surgery, NorthShore University HealthSystem, Evanston, Illinois

Contents

Foreword   xiii

Nicholas J. Petrelli

Preface: Outcomes Research in Surgical Oncology   xv

Clifford Y. Ko and Ryan P. Merkow

Currently Available Quality Improvement Initiatives in Surgical Oncology 367

Ryan P. Merkow and Karl Y. Bilimoria

For most cancers, surgical therapy offers the only hope for cure. Nevertheless, evidence suggests wide variation in cancer care, and therefore it is imperative to ensure that high standards of care are being met. Few initiatives currently exist that are focused on cancer care quality, and there is no program measuring short-term surgical outcomes following cancer surgery. Improvements in care will likely come from performance programs that provide reliable, robust, and actionable information in a timely manner such that performance feedback can occur more frequently and at earlier stages in the treatment and disease process.

Monitoring the Delivery of Cancer Care: Commission on Cancer and National Cancer Data Base   377

Richelle T. Williams, Andrew K. Stewart, and David P. Winchester

The primary objective of the Commission on Cancer (CoC) is to ensure the delivery of comprehensive, high-quality care that improves survival while maintaining quality of life for patients with cancer. This article examines the initiatives of the CoC toward achieving this goal, utilizing data from the National Cancer Data Base (NCDB) to monitor treatment patterns and outcomes, to develop quality measures, and to benchmark hospital performance. The article also highlights how these initiatives align with the Institute of Medicine's recommendations for improving the quality of cancer care and briefly explores future projects of the CoC and NCDB.

Variation in Mortality After High-Risk Cancer Surgery: Failure to Rescue 389

Amir A. Ghaferi and Justin B. Dimick

Surgical mortality with oncologic surgery varies widely in the United States. Patients, providers, and payers are paying closer attention to these variations and a way of reducing them. Although different hospital and surgical technologies and processes of care may account for some of this variation, there is an increasing awareness of the role of hospital safety culture. There is a growing body of evidence suggesting the importance of reducing mortality rates after major complications as a means to reducing the disparate mortality rates with oncologic surgery.

Unexpected Readmissions After Major Cancer Surgery: An Evaluation of Readmissions as a Quality-of-Care Indicator

397

Matthew M. Rochefort and James S. Tomlinson

Readmissions following major oncologic operation are common—affecting patient treatment, outcome, and hospital resources. The Center for Medicare and Medicaid Services mandates reporting of certain disease-specific readmissions and Congress is considering using individual hospital readmission rates as a performance measure. Studies using administrative data demonstrate that readmission rates following major cancer surgery are high. Administrative data cannot determine causes. Single-institution studies demonstrate length of hospital stay and comorbidities as risk factors. Discharge processes and outpatient healthcare utilization can be improved. Until studies on readmission rate are conducted, using readmission rates as a measure of quality should be pursued cautiously.

Importance of and Adherence to Lymph Node Staging Standards in Gastrointestinal Cancer

407

Ryan P. Merkow and David J. Bentrem

In gastrointestinal oncology, one of the most important factors influencing cancer-specific survival is the presence of positive lymph nodes. Although it remains controversial, adequate lymph node examination is required for accurate staging such that patients can receive appropriate adjuvant treatments and for stratification in clinical trials. Nevertheless, wide variation exists in the quality of lymph node examination in the United States, and many centers are not meeting guideline treatment recommendations.

Racial Differences and Disparities in Cancer Care and Outcomes: Where's the Rub?

417

Nestor F. Esnaola and Marvella E. Ford

Despite a profusion of studies over the past several years documenting racial differences in cancer outcomes, there is a paucity of data as to the root causes underlying these observations. This article reviews work to date focusing on black-white differences in cancer outcomes, explores potential mechanisms underlying these differences, and identifies patient, physician, and health care system factors that may account for persistent racial disparities in cancer care. Research strategies to elucidate the relative influence of these various factors and policy recommendations to reduce persistent disparities are also discussed.

Prediction Tools in Surgical Oncology

439

Brandon K. Isariyawongse and Michael W. Kattan

Artificial neural networks, prediction tables, and clinical nomograms allow physicians to transmit an immense amount of prognostic information in a format that exhibits both comprehensibility and brevity. Current models demonstrate that it is feasible to accurately predict many oncologic outcomes, including pathologic stage, recurrence-free survival, and response to adjuvant therapy. Although emphasis should be placed on the independent validation of existing prediction tools, there is a paucity of models in the literature that focus on quality of life outcomes. The unification of tools that predict oncologic and quality of life outcomes into a comparative effectiveness table will furnish patients with cancer with the information they need to make a highly informed and individualized treatment decision.

Randomized Controlled Trials in Surgical Oncology: Where Do We Stand?   449

Kellie L. Mathis and Heidi Nelson

This article reviews the history of clinical trials in surgery using breast cancer surgery and rectal cancer surgery as examples. Trials in breast cancer have transformed the surgical management of this disease. Rectal cancer surgery has also changed greatly, but much of this evolution occurred outside the setting of clinical trials. This article highlights the strengths and limitations of surgical trials and suggests that future studies should include pretrial credentialing as a requirement for surgeon participation. More work needs to be done to bridge the gap from trial results to implementation of new techniques in clinical practice.

Patient Safety in Surgical Oncology: Perspective From the Operating Room   467

Yue-Yung Hu and Caprice C. Greenberg

Despite knowledge that most surgical adverse events occur in the operating room (OR), understanding of the intraoperative phase of care is incomplete; most studies measure surgical safety in terms of preoperative risk or postoperative morbidity and mortality. Because of the OR's complexity, human factors engineering provides an ideal methodology for studies of intraoperative safety. This article reviews models of error and resilience as delineated by human factors experts, correlating them to OR performance. Existing methodologies for studying intraoperative safety are then outlined, focusing on video-based observational research. Finally, specific human and system factors examined in the OR are detailed.

Appropriate Use of Surgical Procedures for Patients with Cancer   479

Elise H. Lawson, Melinda Maggard Gibbons, and Clifford Y. Ko

With increasing focus on improving quality and promoting patient-centered care, ensuring that patients receive appropriate surgical procedures is paramount. The appropriateness method was developed to determine which patients should and should not undergo surgical intervention versus medical therapy. This method combines the best available evidence in the literature with expert opinion to produce explicit guidance for clinicians on the relative risks and benefits of a procedure for specific clinical indications. A coordinated effort to produce appropriateness criteria for surgical oncology could improve the quality of surgical care for patients with cancer if these criteria are integrated into routine clinical practice.

Collaboration with the Community Cancer Center: Benefit for All   487

Nicholas J. Petrelli and Patrick Grusenmeyer

Developing successful programs in a community cancer center involves collaborative efforts between employed and private practice physicians, hospital and cancer center administrations, support personnel, and significant resources, coupled with a vision that will lead to improved patient care and outcomes. Collaboration through a strong state cancer control program is another important component for a successful community cancer center. Delaware has one of the best state cancer control programs in the United States. In 2001, the Delaware Cancer Consortium was formed, which, in 2002, launched its first statewide program to screen all Delawareans older than 50 years with colonoscopy.

Value-Based Health Care: A Surgical Oncologist's Perspective   497

Janice N. Cormier, Kate D. Cromwell, and Raphael E. Pollock

There is ongoing debate on how to reform the health care system. Value-based systems have been proposed to account for both quality and cost. The primary goal of value-based health care is to achieve good health outcomes for patients with consideration of dollars spent. To do so, it is imperative that health care providers define meaningful outcome metrics for specific medical conditions and consider the full cycle of care as well as multiple dimensions of care.

Index   507

SURGICAL ONCOLOGY CLINICS OF NORTH AMERICA

FORTHCOMING ISSUES

October 2012
Laparoscopic Approaches in Oncology
James Fleshman, MD, *Guest Editor*

January 2013
Treatment of Peritoneal Surface Malignancies
Jesus Esquivel, MD, *Guest Editor*

April 2013
Multidisciplinary Care of the Cancer Patient
Greg Masters, MD, *Guest Editor*

RECENT ISSUES

April 2012
Soft Tissue Sarcomas
John M. Kane III, MD, *Guest Editor*

January 2012
Management of Gastric Cancer
Neal Wilkinson, MD, *Guest Editor*

October 2011
Lung Cancer
Mark J. Krasna, MD, *Guest Editor*

NOW AVAILABLE FOR YOUR iPhone and iPad

Foreword

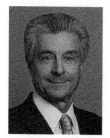

Nicholas J. Petrelli, MD
Consulting Editor

This issue of the *Surgical Oncology Clinics of North America* is devoted to outcomes research in oncology. The guest editor is Clifford Ko, MD, who is Professor of Surgery at UCLA and Director of the UCLA Center for Surgical Outcomes and Quality. Dr Ko's research focuses on studying quality of care, quality of life, and outcomes in cancer surgery, and in view of this, he is an excellent choice as guest editor. No matter what discipline of oncology we center our careers on, it is important that we all develop and improve methods for assessing and monitoring patient-centered care across the cancer continuum. This includes research on patient-centered communication involving cancer patients and survivors, health care delivery teams, and, obviously, family members. The quality of cancer care and the associated health outcomes are an important priority in the United States, especially in view of the rising cost of health care in general.

It is important that we develop interventions that include decision tools for not only clinicians but also patients and the ability to disseminate strategies to move research results rapidly to the provider in the community. The National Cancer Data Base of the Commission on Cancer of the American College of Surgeons is an example of monitoring the delivery of cancer care as explained by Dr David P. Winchester in this edition of the *Surgical Oncology Clinics of North America*. Also, Drs Ghaferi and Dimick from the Center for Health Care Outcomes and Policy at the University of Michigan describe mechanisms underlying variations in hospital mortality rates, which are not well understood. As they explain in their article, *failure to rescue* seems to play an important role in these differences. That is, hospitals with high mortality rates may not be proficient at recognizing and managing serious complications once they occur. This is known as *failure to rescue*. Importantly, progress over the last several decades in cancer treatment, prevention, and control has come from clinical trials. Dr Heidi Nelson from the Mayo Clinic does an excellent job in summarizing where we stand in randomized control trials in surgical oncology.

Last, there are certainly funding opportunities from several of the professional organizations for outcomes research. This includes not only the National Institutes of

Surg Oncol Clin N Am 21 (2012) xiii–xiv
doi:10.1016/j.soc.2012.03.013
1055-3207/12/$ – see front matter

Health, but also the American Society of Clinical Oncology and the American Association for Cancer Research. I'd like to thank Dr Ko and his colleagues for this unique edition of the *Surgical Oncology Clinics of North America*. It is the first time that these *Clinics* have touched on the topic of outcomes research in oncology, which is certainly timely.

Nicholas J. Petrelli, MD
Helen F. Graham Cancer Center
4701 Ogletown-Stanton Road, Suite 1213
Newark, DE 19713, USA

E-mail address:
npetrelli@christianacare.org

Preface

Outcomes Research in Surgical Oncology

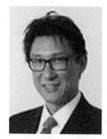

Clifford Y. Ko, MD, MS, MSHS
Guest Editor

Approximately 1.5 million new cancers are diagnosed every year in the United States. Despite improvements in medical therapy, surgical resection remains the only hope for cure and is the primary treatment modality for many of these patients. Countless reports in the past decade have documented wide variation in cancer care quality, and substantial resources have been spent attempting to narrow these treatment gaps. Nevertheless, improving outcomes for any given patient with cancer is a complicated and sometimes monumental endeavor that requires the coordinated effort of all parts of an equally complicated health care system.

In this issue of *Surgical Oncology Clinics of North America*, we sought to highlight many of these efforts, as well as present novel ways to think about and measure cancer care quality, particularly as it relates to surgery. In addition, we aimed to present relevant topics that are broadly applicable to all of surgical oncology, as opposed to focusing on specific disease sites or issues not easily generalizable.

As such, we were extremely fortunate to have leading experts present their work on a variety of diverse topics. The first five articles in this issue relate to the measurement of cancer care quality including current quality initiatives in surgical oncology, monitoring the delivery of cancer care, variation in mortality after high-risk cancer surgery, readmission as a quality indicator, lymph node staging, racial disparities, and the use of prediction tools. The remaining articles are a collage of timely pieces, including the importance of clinical trials in surgical oncology, intraoperative patient safety, appropriateness of cancer care, collaboration with the community cancer center, and value-based cancer care. Although it was not possible to fully capture all aspects of surgical oncology outcomes research, this issue of the *Surgical Oncology Clinics* will hopefully offer a unique perspective that will be both interesting and informative.

Surg Oncol Clin N Am 21 (2012) xv–xvi
doi:10.1016/j.soc.2012.04.001
1055-3207/12/$ – see front matter © 2012 Elsevier Inc. All rights reserved.

surgonc.theclinics.com

Finally, we would like to sincerely thank the authors for their time and effort. Your hard work made this possible. I would also like to thank Nicholas Petrelli for the invitation to put this issue together, and last but not least, his editorial staff for their expertise and support.

Clifford Y. Ko, MD, MS, MSHS
Department of Surgery
University of California, Los Angeles and
VA Greater Los Angeles Healthcare System
10833 LeConte Avenue, 72-215 CHS
Los Angeles, CA 90095, USA

Division of Research and Optimal Patient Care
American College of Surgeons
633 North Saint Clair Street
Chicago, IL 60611, USA

Ryan P. Merkow, MD
Department of Surgery and Surgical Outcomes
and Quality Improvement Center
Northwestern University Feinberg School of Medicine
Chicago, IL, USA

Department of Surgery
University of Colorado School of Medicine
Aurora, CO, USA

Division of Research and Optimal Patient Care
American College of Surgeons
Chicago, IL, USA

E-mail addresses:
CKo@mednet.ucla.edu (C.Y. Ko)
Ryan.Merkow@ucdenver.edu (R.P. Merkow)

Currently Available Quality Improvement Initiatives in Surgical Oncology

Ryan P. Merkow, MD[a,b,c], Karl Y. Bilimoria, MD, MS[d,*]

KEYWORDS

- Quality • Cancer • Quality measure • Surgery • Oncology

KEY POINTS

- For the majority of cancers, surgical therapy offers the only hope for cure. With the aging population and aggressive screening as well as neoadjuvant therapies, increasing numbers of patients will be eligible for surgical resection.
- Evidence suggests wide variation in cancer care quality in the United States.
- Few programs exist that focus on hospital cancer quality, and no program exists that targets hospital surgical quality with respect to short-term outcomes for cancer.
- Improvements in care will likely come from performance programs that provide reliable, robust, and actionable information in a timely manner, such that performance feedback can occur more frequently and at earlier stages in the treatment and disease process.

In 2010, there were approximately 1.5 million new cancer cases diagnosed in the United States, and cancer continued to be the second leading cause of death.[1] Although cancer incidence rates are declining, the overall number of patients diagnosed with a solid organ malignancy is increasing, particularly among the elderly population.[1,2] In addition, broad initiatives have focused on early cancer screening, resulting in an increasing number of patients presenting with early-stage malignancies for which surgical intervention remains the primary treatment modality.[3] Furthermore, with the adoption of more aggressive screening strategies and the increased use of chemoradiotherapy, it is expected that even more patients will be eligible for surgical interventions.[4,5] Therefore, given the growing number of surgeries being performed for cancer, it is imperative to ensure that high standards of care are being met.

[a] Department of Surgery and Surgical Outcomes and Quality Improvement Center, Northwestern University Feinberg School of Medicine, Chicago, IL, USA; [b] Department of Surgery, University of Colorado, School of Medicine, Aurora, CO, USA; [c] Division of Research and Optimal Patient Care, American College of Surgeons, Chicago, IL, USA; [d] Division of Surgical Oncology, Department of Surgery, Institute for Healthcare Studies, Surgical Outcomes and Quality Improvement Center, Northwestern University Feinberg School of Medicine, 676 North Saint Clair Street, Suite 650, Chicago, IL 60611, USA
* Corresponding author.
E-mail address: kbilimoria@nmff.org

Surg Oncol Clin N Am 21 (2012) 367–375
doi:10.1016/j.soc.2012.03.011
1055-3207/12/$ – see front matter © 2012 Elsevier Inc. All rights reserved.
surgonc.theclinics.com

In 1999, the Institute of Medicine (IOM) released its sentinel publication "To Err is Human," which led to an increasing awareness of deficiencies in patient safety in the United States, particularly in surgery.[6] At the same time, the IOM published "Ensuring Quality Cancer Care," which documented substantial variation in the quality of cancer care in the United States.[7] These reports explicitly substantiated the need to consistently and reliably measure the quality of cancer care.

Nevertheless, despite significant effort and cost to develop and improve cancer care, evidence from the ensuing decade suggested that adherence to basic standards of care continued to remain unsatisfactory. For example, in 2003, McGlynn and colleagues[8] documented that only 56% of surgical patients received basic standards of surgical processes of care in the United States. Three years later in 2006, Malin and colleagues[9] evaluated adherence to standards of care in breast and colorectal cancer in 5 metropolitan areas across the United States. They reported an aggregated improvement; however, the variability remained high in certain domains. Specifically, the adherence in breast cancer care was 86% and colorectal cancer 78%, but, in breast cancer, for example, adherence to the 4 surgical quality-of-care measures varied widely from only 30% to nearly 100%.

Although it remains challenging, one approach to reducing this variability in the quality of cancer care is the development, implementation, and feedback of cancer-specific quality measures, such that hospitals can identify areas requiring needed improvements.[10] As such, both governmental and private stakeholders of health care quality have increasingly become intimately involved with cancer care quality improvement specifically around the development of quality improvement initiatives. For example, the National Quality Forum (NQF) launched a program to encourage the development of cancer-specific quality measures, such as ensuring adequate lymph nodes are removed and examined and appropriate postoperative therapies are provided after colectomy for cancer. In addition, recent legislation in the Affordable Care Act provides a clear mandate for performance evaluation, including the requirement of cancer care performance assessment.[11] Also, in late 2010, the Centers for Medicare and Medicaid Services (CMS) announced a contract with 2 private organizations to develop up to 6 cancer-specific quality-of-care measures for eventual use in public reporting. Thus, given the growing attention and importance of quality measurement in surgical oncology, the objectives of this article are (1) to discuss currently available quality measures and initiatives and (2) to explore the specific programs currently available for measuring the quality of cancer care.

DEFINING QUALITY CANCER CARE

The IOM defines quality health care as the "degree to which health services for individuals and populations increase the likelihood of desired health outcomes and are consistent with current professional knowledge."[12] However, defining quality cancer care has proved challenging. Caring for a single patient with cancer requires the coordinated effort of a diverse set of providers and health systems. Traditional definitions of quality measurement use the Donabedian framework of structure, process, and outcomes.[13,14] Structure refers to the system in which the care is delivered such as intensive care unit nurse to patient ratios or presence of interventional radiologists. Processes of care are related to characteristics of the actual care delivered, for example, performing guideline-recommended lymph node examinations or treating patients with stage III colon cancer with adjuvant chemotherapy. Outcomes are often considered the bottom line of quality care; however, there is some debate regarding whether short-term or long-term outcomes should be emphasized.[15] Moreover, measuring outcomes requires rigorous risk adjustment using high-quality data and is heavily dependent on the specific methodology used.[16,17]

Nevertheless, the Donabedian model of quality may not completely encompass the full spectrum of cancer-specific health care quality. Other metrics may be equally or more important. Examples include the accessibility and timeliness of care, cancer-related health care costs, quality-of-life metrics, and the patient centeredness of cancer care. Despite the growing body of knowledge reflecting what constitutes high-quality care, a fundamental challenge lies in determining how to identify poor performance and translate this information into meaningful, real-world changes in clinical practice. The first step may be developing standardized and reliable quality measures and benchmarks of care.

CURRENTLY AVAILABLE CANCER QUALITY MEASURES

Despite the definitional complexity of what constitutes quality cancer care, hospitals and providers must ultimately be evaluated and judged as optimal or in need of improvement. To this end, both private and public organizations, including the NQF, Agency for Healthcare Research and Quality, CMS, the Joint Commission, and the American Hospital Association, have been instrumental in motivating the development of more than 100 measures and benchmarks of care specific to cancer. The NQF has perhaps taken the lead by rigorously and thoroughly evaluating measures based on a set of predefined standards, including clinical importance, scientific acceptability, usability, and feasibility of data collection.[18]

NQF

In 2002, the NQF released an initial call for measures to identify opportunities for health care professionals to improve cancer care. This initiative focused on breast, colorectal, and end-of-life cancer care and resulted in 19 NQF-endorsed performance measures. Breast cancer measures related to surgery included post–breast-conserving surgery irradiation, use of adjuvant chemotherapy or hormone therapy, adherence to the College of American Pathologists Breast Cancer Protocol, use of needle biopsy for diagnosis, and evaluation of axillary lymph nodes in early-stage disease. Colorectal cancer measures included adjuvant chemotherapy use, completeness of pathologic reporting, adherence to the College of American Pathologists Colon and Rectum Protocol, and the examination of at least 12 lymph nodes. Because CMS requires NQF endorsement before their use in public reporting or payment incentives, many of these measures are or will soon be implemented at the national scale.

American Society of Clinical Oncology

In a separate program led by the American Society of Clinical Oncology (ASCO) in conjunction with RAND Corporation and Harvard University, health service researchers conducted the National Initiative on Cancer Care Quality study. Findings from this report identified no surgery-specific measures. Nevertheless, treatment-related measures included optimizing chemotherapy dosing, managing side effects, advising patients about treatment options, better documentation of key cancer staging and treatment details, and ensuring that patients at the highest risk of poor outcomes receive the recommended care.[19]

Other Available Measures

Although most measures reflect breast and colorectal cancers, health services researchers have also identified several quality measures in other cancer sites. In a 2009 study focusing on melanoma care, 26 measures were identified as valid according to RAND/UCLA Appropriateness Methodology.[20] Twenty-four of these measures were processes of care and were mainly related to receiving guideline treatments such as ensuring negative margins, examining appropriate numbers of lymph nodes, and undergoing standard preoperative workup algorithms. A separate report focused on developing pancreatic cancer quality indicators that also used RAND/UCLA Appropriateness Methodology.[21] Forty-three indicators were identified as valid, of which 11 were structural, 19 were process related, 4 addressed treatment appropriateness, 4 assessed efficiency, and 5 assessed outcomes.

Gaps in Cancer Quality Measures

Although many measures have been developed, several gaps exist that need to be addressed. First, of the measures currently available, many are not disease specific or focus only on the most common cancers, such as the NQF-endorsed colorectal and breast cancer quality measures. It should be emphasized that although other cancers are less prevalent, they often have even greater variations in quality. For example, with respect to lymph node examinations following cancer surgery, adherence to the 12–lymph node measure is much better in colon cancer than other common cancers such as esophagus, gastric, and pancreas cancers.[22–24]

Second, there is a lack of surgical outcome assessment in endorsed cancer care quality measures. This is not surprising, given that outcome measures can be considerably more difficult to develop and implement and are at times seen as threatening evaluations. Unlike processes of care, outcomes require the collection of standardized and reliable data for appropriate risk adjustment to account for differences in patient, disease, and procedural risk. Nevertheless, risk-adjusted outcome comparisons may be better reflections of true hospital quality. Recently, the NQF endorsed the first colon resection outcome quality measure, which was developed by the American College of Surgeons (ACS). This measure was demonstrated to be feasible, reliable, and accurate,[25] and, although not intended to be used only after resection for cancer, recent work suggests that cancer-specific variables may not be necessary for robust risk-adjusted hospital quality short-term outcome assessment.[26]

Last, other quality domains that have not been sufficiently addressed include timeliness of care[27] (eg, time from diagnosis to surgery, time for surgical resection to adjuvant chemotherapy in stage III colon cancer) and appropriateness of care[28] (eg, appropriateness of axillary dissection in selected patients with low-risk breast cancer). Nevertheless, these domains are not yet clearly defined, and further research is required before their endorsement and implementation.

Despite the numerous quality indicators currently in existence, without actionable data they cannot affect a meaningful improvement for individual patients with cancer. Nevertheless, it has proved challenging to make this next step, and few programs exist that actually provide this level of data feedback.

PROGRAMS MEASURING CANCER CARE QUALITY

In contrast to the overall number of quality indicators available, the opposite is true of the number of programs that are specifically designed to actually measure provider performance. Nonetheless, a small number of programs exist with the specific aim of improving the quality of surgical care, cancer care, or both.

American Society of Clinical Oncology

The ASCO Quality Oncology Practice Initiative (QOPI) is a unique, multidisciplinary, practice-based, oncologist-run program that began in 2002.[29,30] This program evaluates outpatient oncology practices on a voluntary basis and provides performance feedback to participating providers. QOPI retrospectively reviews charts semi-annually and provides confidential practice-specific comparisons for internal quality improvement purposes. The measures used are all evidence-based quality indicators selected by an expert panel and reassessed every 6 months. At present, there are more than 80 measures being used that range from generalized core measures to metrics specific to breast, colorectal, end-of-life, lymph node, and lung cancers. Practices can obtain QOPI certification based on compliance with oncology-specific standards and sufficient performance with respect to quality metrics. This program currently has more than 700 participating practices across the Unites States. Nevertheless, this program generally reflects outpatient cancer care indicators, and does not directly assess surgical quality.

Commission on Cancer

The longest standing program establishing cancer care quality standards is the Commission on Cancer (CoC).[31] The CoC was established by the ACS in the first part of the twentieth century, and, at present, more than 1500 cancer centers are accredited by this organization, accounting for more than 70% of all newly diagnosed malignancies in the United States. However, the CoC is more than an accreditation program. Two new initiatives, the Cancer Program Practice Profile Reports (CP3R) and the Rapid Quality Reporting System (RQRS), are currently available to provide cancer centers with actionable performance feedback based on endorsed standards.[32]

The CP3R initiative focuses on colorectal and breast cancers by using the NQF-endorsed quality measures to assess hospital level performance across CoC sites.[33] The data collection process uses the National Cancer Data Base, and, after hospitals are audited to ensure the completeness of their data, programs can receive detailed reports reflecting their performance, compared with those of other hospitals. At present, this is the only program that provides cancer-specific feedback to cancer centers.

A second CoC endeavor, RQRS, was specifically developed to provide more immediate performance feedback to participating hospitals by simultaneously collecting and reporting patient data. This way, individual patients will experience evidence-based real-time quality improvements. This program also focuses on the NQF-endorsed measures and generates alerts if the expected treatment is not reported within a prespecified time frame. Both the registry staff and program leadership receive these alerts and report this information to the specific caregivers who can ensure that the appropriate treatments are being provided. In addition to the alert mechanism, the system has an online dashboard specific to each program, such that individual patients can be identified and receipt of guideline treatments tracked over time.

National Surgical Quality Improvement Program

For hospital-level performance measurement to be trusted, it must have an accurate, reliable, and standardized data collection process. Although the ACS National Surgical Quality Improvement Program (NSQIP) is not a cancer-specific platform, it is the clear leader in data collection, measurement, and outcome performance feedback in surgery. Beginning in the Veterans Affairs system in 1994, NSQIP was integrated into the private sector in 2001 and began providing hospital level performance reports to hospitals in 2005. Since that time it has demonstrated to be reliable,[34] to improve hospital performance in the majority of participating hospitals,[35] and to reduce health care costs.[36]

Nevertheless, ACS NSQIP historically has not compiled procedure-specific data, which has long been an important goal of the program.[37] To address these interests, a program was recently developed that allows hospitals to choose from 34 specific procedures, including pancreatectomy, hepatectomy, colectomy, proctectomy, esophagectomy, and lung resection. In addition, each procedure includes a set of customized process-related and outcome-specific variables, selected by leading national experts and specialty societies. Many of these procedures include cancer-specific variables. For example, pancreatectomy includes an outcome variable for pancreatic leak, and participating hospitals are able to evaluate their risk-adjusted hospital performance with respect to this outcome, compared with other ACS NSQIP hospitals.

Other cancer-related variables specific to pancreatectomy include preoperative obstructive jaundice, preoperative biliary stent, vascular resection performed, type of pancreatic reconstruction, placement of operative drains, American Joint Committee on Cancer (AJCC) stage, and delayed gastric emptying. Likewise, colon and rectum operations have cancer-related, process-related, and outcome variables, including AJCC stage, surgical margin status, tumor size and number of lymph nodes examined, prolonged postoperative ileus, and anastomotic leak. Other unique cancer-specific variable examples include use of preoperative positron emission tomographic scans in esophageal cancer and use of concurrent intraoperative ablation during hepatectomy.

Although the contribution of the Procedure Targeted program to the measurement of surgical quality is remarkable, the program still provides hospitals with reports that include all patients irrespective of operative indication (eg, cancer status). This may lead to a void for cancer centers and hospitals that want to separately examine their cancer surgery care as their casemix is not uniquely represented in the currently available ACS NSQIP reports. Moreover, there are no robust initiatives that allow hospitals to assess the quality of their surgical cancer care. To this end, the ACS NSQIP is currently developing an oncology-specific consortium, the Oncology NSQIP National Cancer Institute Center Consortium, to specifically address this need. The objectives of this initiative are to provide hospitals with cancer-specific comparative outcomes, test and develop new variables and outcomes, and develop the best practice guidelines of surgical oncology. In a recent feasibility project, the authors found wide variation in cancer-specific risk-adjusted outcomes, even among National Cancer

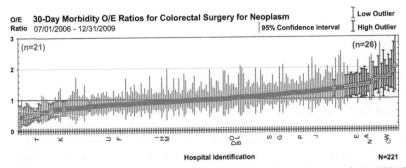

Fig. 1. Risk-adjusted hospital comparisons after colorectal surgery for cancer from ACS NSQIP (2006–2009). Each letter denotes a National Cancer Institute hospital. O/E and 95% confidence interval <1.0 denotes performance better than expected. O/E and 95% confidence interval >1.0 denotes performance worse than expected.

Institute hospitals (**Fig. 1**), further emphasizing the need for cancer-specific quality improvement initiatives.

FUTURE DIRECTIONS

As payers, purchasers, and consumers of health care increasingly focus on quality measurement and improvement, providers will certainly be held accountable for the care that is delivered, and this information will be made available to the public. These issues are especially relevant to the oncology community in which considerable variation exists in the quality of care. Moreover, with the growing complexity of screening, diagnosis, and cancer treatments, the importance of benchmarking performance will continue to grow. To ensure high-quality care, both private and public organizations must continue to support the development of important, reliable, and feasibly collected quality measures as well as continue to support quality improvement programs. In step with the Commission on Cancer's Rapid Reporting System, performance feedback should ideally occur more frequently and at earlier stages in the treatment and disease process, such that actionable quality improvements can be made at the individual patient level.

SUMMARY

Improving the quality of cancer care is a complex, difficult, yet necessary endeavor. As the prevalence of Americans living with cancer increases and more individuals are candidates for surgical treatments, it is essential to continue to develop, measure, implement, and provide high-quality real-time feedback on provider performance. Several quality measures in cancer care exist; however, there is a continued need for disease site–specific metrics with greater emphasis on surgical treatment. More importantly, the currently available measures must be appropriately implemented to affect meaningful change. Local, regional, and national organizations must continue to support quality improvement initiatives, so that all patients receive evidence-based high-quality cancer-directed care.

REFERENCES

1. Jemal A, Siegel R, Xu J, et al. Cancer statistics, 2010. CA Cancer J Clin 2010; 60(5):277–300.
2. Yancik R, Ries LA. Aging and cancer in America. Demographic and epidemiologic perspectives. Hematol Oncol Clin North Am 2000;14(1):17–23.
3. Gross CP, Andersen MS, Krumholz HM, et al. Relation between Medicare screening reimbursement and stage at diagnosis for older patients with colon cancer. JAMA 2006;296(23):2815–22.
4. Merkow RP, Bilimoria KY, McCarter MD, et al. Use of multimodality neoadjuvant therapy for esophageal cancer in the United States: assessment of 987 hospitals. Ann Surg Oncol 2012;19(2):357–64.
5. Bilimoria KY, Bentrem DJ, Ko CY, et al. Multimodality therapy for pancreatic cancer in the U.S.: utilization, outcomes, and the effect of hospital volume. Cancer 2007; 110(6):1227–34.
6. Kohn L, Corrigan J, Donaldson M, editors. To err is human: building a safer health system. Washington, DC: Committee on Quality of Health Care in America, Institute of Medicine. National Academies Press; 1999.

7. Hewitt M, Simone JV, editors. Ensuring quality cancer care. Washington, DC: Institute of Medicine, Commission on Life Sciences, National Cancer Policy Board and National Research Council. National Academy Press; 1999.
8. McGlynn EA, Asch SM, Adams J, et al. The quality of health care delivered to adults in the United States. N Engl J Med 2003;348(26):2635–45.
9. Malin JL, Schneider EC, Epstein AM, et al. Results of the National Initiative for Cancer Care Quality: how can we improve the quality of cancer care in the United States? J Clin Oncol 2006;24(4):626–34.
10. Institute of Medicine. Performance measurement: accelerating improvement-pathways to quality health care series. Washington, DC: National Academies Press; 2006.
11. Affordable Care Act (ACA): Sec. 3005. Quality reporting for PPS-exempt cancer hospitals. Available at: http://healthreformgps.org/wp-content/uploads/Medicare-Provisions-in-the-ACA-Summary-and-Timeline.pdf. Accessed August 20, 2011.
12. Institute of Medicine of the National Academies. A National Clinical Trials System for the 21st century: reinvigorating the NCI Cooperative Group Program. Available at: http://www.iom.edu/Reports/2010/A-National-Cancer-Clinical-Trials-System-for-the-21st-Century-Reinvigorating-the-NCI-Cooperative.aspx. Accessed June 24, 2011.
13. Donabedian A. The quality of care. How can it be assessed? JAMA 1988;260(12): 1743–8.
14. Birkmeyer JD, Dimick JB, Birkmeyer NJ. Measuring the quality of surgical care: structure, process, or outcomes? J Am Coll Surg 2004;198(4):626–32.
15. Bilimoria KY, Bentrem DJ, Feinglass JM, et al. Directing surgical quality improvement initiatives: comparison of perioperative mortality and long-term survival for cancer surgery. J Clin Oncol 2008;26(28):4626–33.
16. Shahian DM, Wolf RE, Iezzoni LI, et al. Variability in the measurement of hospital-wide mortality rates. N Engl J Med 2010;363(26):2530–9.
17. Bilimoria KY, Cohen ME, Merkow RP, et al. Comparison of outlier identification methods in hospital surgical quality improvement programs. J Gastrointest Surg 2010;14(10):1600–7.
18. The National Quality Forum (NQF). Available at: http://www.qualityforum.org/Home.aspx. Accessed August 1, 2011.
19. American Society of Clinical Oncology. National Initiative on Cancer Care Quality (NICCQ). Available at: http://www.asco.org/ASCOv2/Practice+%26+Guidelines/Quality+Care/Quality+Measurement+%26+Improvement/NICCQ. Accessed August 15, 2011.
20. Bilimoria KY, Raval MV, Bentrem DJ, et al. National assessment of melanoma care using formally developed quality indicators. J Clin Oncol 2009;27(32):5445–51.
21. Bilimoria KY, Bentrem DJ, Lillemoe KD, et al. Assessment of pancreatic cancer care in the United States based on formally developed quality indicators. J Natl Cancer Inst 2009;101(12):848–59.
22. Merkow RP, Bilimoria KY, Chow WB, et al. Variation in lymph node examination after esophagectomy for cancer in the United States. Arch Surg 2012. [Epub ahead of print].
23. Bilimoria KY, Talamonti MS, Wayne JD, et al. Effect of hospital type and volume on lymph node evaluation for gastric and pancreatic cancer. Arch Surg 2008;143(7): 671–8 [discussion: 678].
24. Bilimoria KY, Bentrem DJ, Stewart AK, et al. Lymph node evaluation as a colon cancer quality measure: a national hospital report card. J Natl Cancer Inst 2008; 100(18):1310–7.

25. Merkow RP, Hall BL, Cohen ME, et al. Validity and feasibility of the American College of Surgeons Colectomy Composite Outcome Quality Measure. Ann Surg, in press.
26. Merkow RP, Kmiecik TE, Bentrem DL, et al. The importance of cancer-specific variables in risk-adjusted hospital quality comparisons for ACS NSQIP short-term outcomes. Presented at the Society of Surgical Oncology 65th Cancer Symposium. Orlando (FL), 2012.
27. Bilimoria KY, Ko CY, Tomlinson JS, et al. Wait times for cancer surgery in the United States: trends and predictors of delays. Ann Surg 2011;253(4):779–85.
28. Lee CN, Ko CY. Beyond outcomes—the appropriateness of surgical care. JAMA 2009;302(14):1580–1.
29. Neuss MN, Desch CE, McNiff KK, et al. A process for measuring the quality of cancer care: the Quality Oncology Practice Initiative. J Clin Oncol 2005;23(25): 6233–9.
30. American Society of Clinical Oncology. The Quality Oncology Practice Initiative. Available at: http://qopi.asco.org/program. Accessed August 25, 2011.
31. The American College of Surgeons, Cancer Programs. The Commission on Cancer. Available at: http://www.facs.org/cancer/coc/cocar.html. Accessed August 15, 2011.
32. Raval MV, Bilimoria KY, Stewart AK, et al. Using the NCDB for cancer care improvement: an introduction to available quality assessment tools. J Surg Oncol 2009;99(8):488–90.
33. American College of Surgeons, Cancer Programs. CoC Quality Care Measures. Available at: http://www.facs.org/cancer/qualitymeasures.html. Accessed August 15, 2011.
34. Shiloach M, Frencher SK Jr, Steeger JE, et al. Toward robust information: data quality and inter-rater reliability in the American College of Surgeons National Surgical Quality Improvement Program. J Am Coll Surg 2010;210(1):6–16.
35. Hall BL, Hamilton BH, Richards K, et al. Does surgical quality improve in the American College of Surgeons National Surgical Quality Improvement Program: an evaluation of all participating hospitals. Ann Surg 2009;250(3):363–76.
36. Dimick JB, Chen SL, Taheri PA, et al. Hospital costs associated with surgical complications: a report from the private-sector National Surgical Quality Improvement Program. J Am Coll Surg 2004;199(4):531–7.
37. Birkmeyer JD, Shahian DM, Dimick JB, et al. Blueprint for a new American College of Surgeons: National Surgical Quality Improvement Program. J Am Coll Surg 2008;207(5):777–82.

Monitoring the Delivery of Cancer Care
Commission on Cancer and National Cancer Data Base

Richelle T. Williams, MD[a,b], Andrew K. Stewart, MA[b],
David P. Winchester, MD[b,c],*

KEYWORDS

- Quality • Cancer • Registry • Commission on cancer • National Cancer Data Base

KEY POINTS

- Cancer is an important part of any discussion about quality because of the complexity of treatment and disproportionate cost of caring for these patients.
- The National Cancer Data Base (NCDB) plays a central role in the Commission on Cancer's (CoC's) efforts to ensure the delivery of high-quality cancer care.
- NCDB data affect patient care through two major pathways: hospital benchmarking with resultant quality improvement initiatives and research to develop new quality measures.
- The Rapid Quality Reporting System is a novel online NCDB tool that changes the cancer data paradigm by assessing compliance with treatment standards in real time.
- Increasing patient-centered care and incorporating patient-reported outcomes represent key next steps by the CoC and NCDB to enhance cancer care.

Health care is changing rapidly, with health reform currently at the forefront and cost containment an imperative that can no longer be ignored. Although cancer is not the most common disease affecting Americans, it accounts for a disproportionate fraction of the cost of health care in the United States and is, therefore, an extremely important topic in the current health care environment.[1,2] Fortunately, discussions around access, quality, and cost are not new to oncology and really came to the fore in 1999

The authors have no relevant disclosures.
[a] Department of Surgery, University of Chicago Medical Center 5841 South, Maryland Avenue, Chicago, IL 60637, USA; [b] Cancer Programs, American College of Surgeons, 633 North Saint Clair Street, Chicago, IL 60611-3211, USA; [c] Department of Surgery, NorthShore University HealthSystem, Evanston Hospital, 2650 Ridge Avenue, Evanston, IL 60201, USA
* Corresponding author. Cancer Programs, American College of Surgeons, 633 North Saint Clair Street, Chicago, IL 60611-3211.
E-mail address: dwinchester@northshore.org

Surg Oncol Clin N Am 21 (2012) 377–388
doi:10.1016/j.soc.2012.03.005
1055-3207/12/$ – see front matter © 2012 Elsevier Inc. All rights reserved.

when the Institute of Medicine's (IOM's) National Cancer Policy Board called for improved delivery and quality of cancer care.[3]

In its follow-up report in 2000, the IOM advocated for the enhancement of cancer care data systems through several mechanisms as one of the essential steps toward ensuring quality cancer care.[4] These mechanisms included (paraphrased from Part 1 of the recommendations):

- Identification and inclusion of a core set of evidence-based quality measures
- Standardization of reporting, especially with regard to disease stage and patient comorbidity
- Linkage to other data sources (such as administrative data) and special studies to give a more rounded picture of the continuum of cancer care as well as provide the necessary data elements for case-mix adjustment in studies comparing care in one setting versus another
- Reporting quality benchmarks and performance data to institutions giving care to patients with cancer
- Information technology solutions to increase coverage, quality, and timely availability of relevant clinical data
- Training of health service researchers with special emphasis on implementation of quality improvement initiatives and measurement of quality of care.

This report also cited the Commission on Cancer's (CoC's) National Cancer Data Base (NCDB) as one of the most promising cancer data systems for affecting quality.

With this backdrop and the understanding that the core mission of the CoC and NCDB is improving the quality of cancer care, the remainder of this article proceeds as follows. First, it describes the structure and organization of the NCDB and examines where the NCDB fits within the larger picture of central cancer registries. Next, it addresses the several mechanisms for enhancing cancer care data systems put forth by the IOM and highlights the ways in which the CoC and NCDB have answered the call either via completed projects or works in progress. In each case, stumbling blocks during implementation and/or limitations will be noted. Finally, it provides a sense of the direction and vision of the CoC and NCDB for impacting and improving cancer care going forward.

NCDB-CANCER REGISTRY STRUCTURE AND ORGANIZATION

The NCDB is a joint program of the American College of Surgeons' CoC and the American Cancer Society and is one of three main cancer registry systems in the country. The other two programs are the Centers for Disease Control and Prevention's National Program of Cancer Registries (NPCR) and the National Cancer Institute's (NCI's) Surveillance, Epidemiology, and End Results (SEER) program. The NPCR receives information on new cancer cases from virtually every state through the system of state cancer registries. This system capitalizes on the fact that cancer is a reportable disease and, therefore, captures an estimated 96% of the United States population.[5] In comparison, SEER collects data from regions in 15 states using complex sampling methods and represents about 28% of the population.[6] In contrast to the NPCR and SEER programs, which are both population-based, the NCDB is a hospital-based registry that includes cases from approximately 1500 CoC-accredited institutions nationwide and currently accounts for approximately 70% of cancers diagnosed in the United States.[7]

Although the NCDB is hospital-based, because of its fairly large footprint NCDB data can be reasonably extrapolated to the population for many tumor sites, with a few important caveats. Compared to non–CoC-approved hospitals in the United States, CoC hospitals are more likely to be teaching or research hospitals.[8] Although three-quarters of hospitals participating in the CoC accreditation program are community-based centers and account for approximately 60% of the cases reported to the NCDB, teaching or research centers make up a fifth of all CoC-accredited programs and more than a third of the cases reported to the NCDB on an annual basis (**Table 1**). This has possible implications for the generalizability of NCDB data. In addition, tumors that are much less likely to require hospitalization for treatment (eg, early-stage melanoma and prostate cancer) are proportionally underrepresented in the NCDB.[9] Furthermore, there can be significant differences by region due to variable penetrance of CoC accreditation. In 2006, the distribution of CoC-approved institutions by state ranged from 0% in Wyoming to 100% in Delaware.[8] A comparison of NCDB and state registry data between 2003 and 2007 for 28 states demonstrated that the proportion of all cancer cases captured in the NCDB was as low as 27.2% in Arizona to as high as 90.0% in North Dakota (Anthony S. Robbins, MD, PhD, American Cancer Society, personal communication, 2012).

The NCDB processes data on over one million cancer cases annually and contains information on almost 28 million cases in total since 1985. Registrars report specific data elements that include patient demographics (age, sex, race/ethnicity, payer information), cancer stage (clinical and pathologic), tumor characteristics (including histology, grade, site-specific prognostic factors), first-course therapy (type of surgery, type and extent of radiation, chemotherapy, immunotherapy, and hormone therapy), and outcomes (surgical margin status, recurrence, and survival). Several of these data items are common across all three registry systems, but a few are unique to NCDB data—notably *International Classification of Diseases, 9th and 10th edition, Clinical Modification* (ICD-9/10-CM) codes for comorbid diagnoses and detailed radiation modality and dosing information.[10] Data are collected in accordance with nationally standardized procedures and reporting formats coordinated by the North American Association of Central Cancer Registries (NAACCR), the collaborative umbrella organization for all central cancer registries in the United States and Canada.[11] Data reported to the NCDB are then linked to tertiary data sources (facility and census data) to provide hospital characteristics and area-based socioeconomic indicators, such as income and education.[7,9] These data are processed and fed back to the reporting hospitals so they can assess the performance of their cancer program either on its own or compared to other programs. This is achieved through a variety of online tools (see later discussion).

Monitoring and Improving Cancer Care Through Enhanced Data Systems

Before delving into each of the mechanisms proposed by the IOM and the response of the CoC and NCDB, it is useful to have a conceptual framework for how the CoC seeks

Table 1
Distribution of cancer programs and cases in the NCDB (2008)

Cancer Program Type	As a % of CoC-Accredited Programs	As a % of Cases Reported to NCDB
Small community	33	14
Comprehensive community	42	48
Academic	17	26
NCI-designated	2	9
Veterans Affairs (VA)	4	3
—	n = 1500	n ≈ 1.1 million

to affect quality-of-care using cancer registry data. For simplicity, NCDB data may be viewed as affecting patient care through two major pathways: (1) benchmarking and the resultant quality improvement initiatives with respect to established standards and (2) research to develop new quality metrics (**Fig. 1**).

Evidence-based cancer care quality measures

The classic paradigm for assessing health care was defined by Donabedian[12] and divides quality measures into three main types: structure, process, and outcome. Structure refers to the attributes of the system in which care is delivered (eg, the number of hospital beds or the presence of an electronic health record). Process measures encompass the interactions between the providers and patients in the actual delivery of health care. An example might be whether an eligible patient received appropriate chemotherapy for their cancer. Outcomes are those changes in health status that are attributable to the health care received, such as mortality or rates of surgical-site infections.

An alternative approach, which perhaps has a more administrative and/or surveillance focus, classifies quality measures based on their potential utilization. With this approach, measures are divided into (1) accountability measures, which are supported by data from randomized controlled trials and can be used for public reporting and payment incentive programs; (2) quality improvement measures, supported by evidence from retrospective studies and used for internal monitoring of performance; and (3) surveillance measures, supported by consensus expert opinion and used to monitor patterns of care and guide policymaking.[13,14] This framework is the one used by the National Quality Forum (NQF) and therefore provides the terminology adopted by the CoC in its process of measure development.

The CoC screens and evaluates potential measures using the four domains used by the NQF[15]:

1. *Importance.* Measures are accompanied by a full literature review of trials or relevant meta-analyses, with a corresponding evaluation of how the measure relates to outcomes and clinical practice guidelines. This also provides the rationale for whether the measure should be described as an accountability, quality improvement, or surveillance measure. Each measure includes an estimate of the number of cancer cases potentially affected and describes any anticipated sensitivity or variance issues associated with the measure.

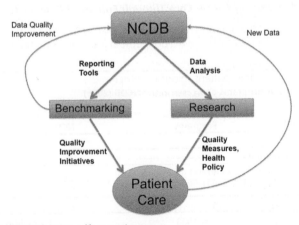

Fig. 1. Using registry data to affect patient care.

2. *Scientific acceptability*. Measures are well defined, precisely specified, and adaptable to patient preferences. They can be regularly applied with consistent results that adequately discriminate between real differences in provider behavior. When a risk-adjustment strategy is necessary, this is also described.
3. *Usability*. Measures can be used for assessing programmatic performance, making decisions, and implementing change.
4. *Feasibility*. The relative ease or burden of data collection is considered. Data collection should be clearly associated with the delivery of care and obtained within the normal flow of clinical care.

The NCDB's reliance on data reported from hospital cancer registries is the central limiting factor shaping these particular discussions. For example, measures cannot be defined around administration of a particular therapeutic drug at this time because specific drugs are not identified in the registry. Confidentiality and audit requirements are also important considerations.

In 2005, as part of the response to the IOM report, the NQF initiated a call for evidence-based cancer quality measures. In a joint effort with the National Comprehensive Cancer Network (NCCN) and the American Society of Clinical Oncology (ASCO), the CoC developed six measures for breast and colorectal cancer care.[16] Five of these measures were endorsed by the NQF in 2007 (**Table 2**). These quality

Table 2	
Cancer quality measures	
Organ Site	**Measure**
Breast	Radiation therapy is administered within 1 year (365 d) of diagnosis for women under age 70 receiving breast conserving surgery for breast cancer[a]
	Combination chemotherapy is considered or administered within 4 months (120 d) of diagnosis for women under 70 with AJCC T1cN0M0, or stage II or III hormone receptor negative breast cancer[a]
	Tamoxifen or third generation aromatase inhibitor is considered or administered within 1 year (365 d) of diagnosis for women with AJCC T1cN0M0, or stage II or III hormone receptor positive breast cancer[a]
	Core needle or FNA biopsy is performed before surgical treatment of breast cancer[b]
	Breast conservation surgery rate for women with AJCC stage 0, I or II breast cancer[b]
	Radiation therapy is considered or administered within 1 year (365 d) of diagnosis for women undergoing mastectomy for breast cancer with 4 or more positive regional lymph nodes[b]
Colon	At least 12 regional lymph nodes are removed and pathologically examined for resected colon cancer[a]
	Adjuvant chemotherapy is considered or administered within 4 months (120 d) of diagnosis for patients under the age of 80 with AJCC stage III (lymph node positive) colon cancer[a]
Rectum	Radiation therapy is considered or administered within 6 months (180 d) of diagnosis for patients under the age of 80 with clinical or pathologic AJCC T4N0M0 or stage III disease receiving surgical resection for rectal cancer

Abbreviations: AJCC, American Joint Committee on Cancer; FNA, fine-needle aspiration.
 [a] NQF-endorsed measures. All measures except the 12-regional-nodes measure for colon were endorsed as accountability measures the 12-node measure was endorsed as a quality-improvement measure.
 [b] Breast measures in bold represent the new CoC-approved quality measures of 2011.

measures have all been widely adopted and compliance rates are now actively monitored in cancer programs across the country.

The CoC has continued work to identify and specify additional quality measures, placing an early emphasis on breast, upper gastrointestinal, and lung cancers, with the goal of introducing hospital-level quality improvement measures that can be supported through the NCDB. Measures are reviewed for several characteristics, including validity, reliability, feasibility, and whether they are evidence-based and the results are actionable and usable at the local level by CoC-accredited cancer programs. These efforts leverage the collaborative relationships that the CoC maintains with its member organizations, professional medical societies, clinical trials cooperative groups (eg, the newly formed Alliance), and other agencies focused on the development and implementation of cancer-related quality measures. To the extent possible, the specification of potential measures is kept in step with frameworks, priorities, and goals established by organizations already engaged in measure development, assessment, and endorsement. So far, in 2011, three additional breast cancer measures have been adopted (see **Table 2**) and these will be incorporated into the CoC's core group of quality measures going forward.

Standardization of reporting

In addition to a core set of quality indicators, efforts to evaluate and improve cancer care require standardized measures of cancer stage and patient comorbidity. This ensures that comparisons are made across equivalent groups of patients and differences can then be more confidently attributed to the quality of health care received. The best example of attempts to unify registry staging data is Collaborative Stage (CS), a project sponsored by the American Joint Committee on Cancer (AJCC) in collaboration with the CoC, SEER, NPCR, NAACCR, the National Cancer Registrars Association, and the Canadian Cancer Society.[17] The initial goal was to develop a system with an ability to translate between the two registry staging schema, AJCC TNM stage and SEER summary stage. This would, hopefully ease the burden on registrars of duplicate abstraction to accommodate the different staging systems. CS, which has been applied to cases from 2004 onward, was designed to use all the available information to derive a single, best stage for any given patient. By coding additional site-specific details about the extent of disease, CS should in theory increase portability across time by bridging changes in stage definitions. There is also the significant benefit of providing a way to quickly add relevant, nonanatomic, site-specific prognostic factors to cancer registry data. For example, human epidermal growth factor receptor 2 (HER2/neu) status in breast cancer will be collected as a CS site-specific factor starting with cases diagnosed in 2010. One shortcoming of this approach is that clinical stage is not clearly delineated in this final best stage. This has become more important as the use of neoadjuvant therapy has increased. In this regard, the separate clinical and pathologic TNM staging collected in the NCDB are key in monitoring appropriate utilization of the different therapeutic options for a given tumor.

Case mix adjustment is also pivotal in any comparative assessment of quality and outcomes. Recognizing this, the NCDB began to collect ICD-9-CM secondary diagnoses codes in 2003 to derive comorbidity scores that can be used in the adjustment for comorbid disease burden in its analyses. As mentioned previously, among the three main cancer registries in the United States, this data item is unique to the NCDB. Currently, both Charlson-Dayo and Elixhauser comorbidity measures are available in the dataset. Although either comorbidity score used in combination with race/ethnicity, age, sex, and stage is still an imperfect adjustment for case mix, it represents a definite improvement.

Linkage to other data sources and special studies

The CoC's and NCDB's quality improvement initiatives also require access to complete treatment information. Although cancer registries are a key source of this information, they have long been viewed with suspicion regarding the completeness of the data captured and reported. Because registries are primarily hospital-based, they have difficulty identifying all chemotherapy, endocrine therapy, and radiation administered in the outpatient setting. Previous studies, primarily reflecting registry operations in the 1990s, showed that, for breast and colorectal cancer, registries captured as little as 70% of administered chemotherapy, 60% of radiation, and 50% to 60% of endocrine treatment.[18] More recently, a study lead by investigators from the NPCR program reported on the quality and completeness of data reported for breast and prostate cancer cases. Although differences in study methodology limit direct comparisons with earlier efforts, the results from their re-abstracting study suggest that reliability and completeness of treatment information captured by cancer registries has improved over time. The sensitivity of surgery information improved from 92% (between 1997 and 1998) to 98% (between 2007 and 2009). Radiation increased from 74% to 88%, chemotherapy from 71% to 75%, and hormone therapy from 49% to 69%.[19]

Obtaining truly complete registry data would require additional sources of information to supplement the existing data or call for large-scale record re-abstraction. The latter is logistically difficult and prohibitively expensive. Alternatively, administrative or claims data collected by insurance payers are a recognized complement to registry data. Claims data provide information on all medical services received by a patient regardless of treatment venue. However, alone, they are of limited value in evaluating cancer care because information about the date of cancer diagnosis and cancer stage is absent. Linking claims and registry data provides a robust tool for quality evaluation. The utility of this approach has been demonstrated by linkage of the NCI's SEER data to fee-for-service Medicare claims. The SEER-Medicare linked file has been widely used for study of care of older Americans who reside in the SEER regions.[20] Capitalizing on this paradigm, the NCDB has collaborated with two private payers to assess the completeness of registry data across 3 years (2004–2006) for breast and colorectal cancers diagnosed among residents of Ohio. This was achieved by linking claims data from United HealthCare and Anthem Blue Cross-Blue Shield of Ohio to the NCDB and the Ohio Cancer Incidence Surveillance System, the state cancer registry in Ohio (Malin and colleagues, unpublished material, 2011). Preliminary results of this work show that treatment information in registries remains incomplete, but not nearly to the extent described by Malin and colleagues, capturing as much as 87% of administered chemotherapy, 86% of radiation, and 64% of endocrine treatment for breast and colorectal cancers.

One final avenue for enriching registry data that is worth mentioning is via NCDB special studies. These have typically been used for relatively rare tumors, where the sample size is fairly small, or for a specific subset of patients with more common tumors, where appropriate sampling methods can be used to minimize the burden of data collection while ensuring sufficient power to support the proposed analysis. For these studies, registrars are asked to submit information not ordinarily available in registry data from the medical records of patients identified in the NCDB, such as clinical presentation, imaging data or the names of specific drugs used for treatment. Special studies are an invaluable adjunct to NCDB data because they provide an opportunity to answer research questions that require detailed clinical information not routinely found in registries. However, the burden of data collection for registrars can be substantial, and the predicted impact of the study findings relative to this burden is one of the main considerations in the CoC's approval process for these studies.

Quality benchmarks and performance data

Acknowledging the limitations of registry data and the need for complete data for quality analysis, the NCDB has implemented retrospective and prospective audit and reporting tools such as the Cancer Program Practice Profile Reports (CP³R) and Rapid Quality Reporting System (RQRS) that have lead to changes in registry operations that both enhance data quality and improve patient care. The CP³R has been available to CoC-accredited cancer programs since 2005 and it provides programs the ability to review and compare their performance on specific clinical process measures with other programs locally, regionally, and nationally.[21] A specific feature of the CP³R is that cancer programs have the ability to review case-level concordance with applicable measures and to update incomplete or under-reported treatment information. Programs that engage in this level of review and reconciliation generally demonstrate significantly improved performance rates of as much as 15% to 20% (unpublished data from the NCDB, 2010), suggesting that adjuvant or ambulatory treatment information is available to registries when the context of and incentive for chart reviews is specifically defined.

Stemming from examination of CP³R compliance rates in their institution between 2004 and 2007 for the colon and rectal cancer quality measures (see **Table 2**), Pappas and colleagues[22] described the development of two quality improvement initiatives that would directly affect patient care: pretreatment staging with MRI for patients with rectal cancer to delineate those appropriate for neoadjuvant radiation and a colon cancer protocol to ensure a thorough search for 12 lymph nodes. In another study, Lodrigues and colleagues[23] performed medical record audits to investigate why their institution's compliance rates in 2004 for the three NQF-endorsed breast cancer measures included in CP³R (see **Table 2**) were lower than expected (21%, 26%, and 61% for the hormonal therapy, radiation, and chemotherapy measures, respectively). After reviewing the relevant records, their recalculated compliance rates were 88% for hormonal therapy, 98% for radiation therapy, and 97% for chemotherapy. The discrepancy was due to a combination of poor physician documentation and treatment records that were not accessible by their tumor registry staff. This cancer program has since addressed both issues, resulting in a marked improvement in the quality of their registry data.

Increasing coverage, quality, and timeliness of data

Perhaps one of the biggest limitations of registry data is that data are typically not available for analysis and reporting until up to 2 years following the initial diagnosis, a reflection of the time required to abstract and report individual cases to centralized data repositories and subsequently to process and aggregate large data sets. Although these retrospective data remain quite valuable for benchmarking and quality improvement efforts such as those described in the previous section, it is often too late to affect the care of the patients represented in the dataset. More recently, the NCDB has released the RQRS, a quality improvement tool that provides real-time assessment of hospital adherence to NQF-endorsed quality-of-cancer-care measures.[24] In contrast to the retrospective CP³R that provides an assessment of clinical performance based on past practices, the RQRS facilitates continuous quality improvement and enables CoC-accredited cancer programs to report data on patients concurrently. RQRS actively alerts hospitals about outstanding treatment, thereby promoting a continuous review of local processes of care while patients are still engaged in the treatment of their disease (**Fig. 2**A). RQRS also provides hospitals with year-to-date concordance rates relative to other programs at the state and national level (**Fig. 2**B).

Because of these characteristics, RQRS has played an important part in a large-scale project to develop a rapid learning system for cancer in the state of Georgia, with the 30 participating CoC programs in Georgia making up a large fraction of the 65 total beta test sites for RQRS.[25] As of summer 2011, beta testing has been completed and RQRS is now available to all CoC-accredited programs on a volunteer basis.

Training of health service researchers
The final mechanism outlined in the IOM report was the "training of professionals with expertise in the measurement of quality of care...".[4] In 2005, the CoC began the

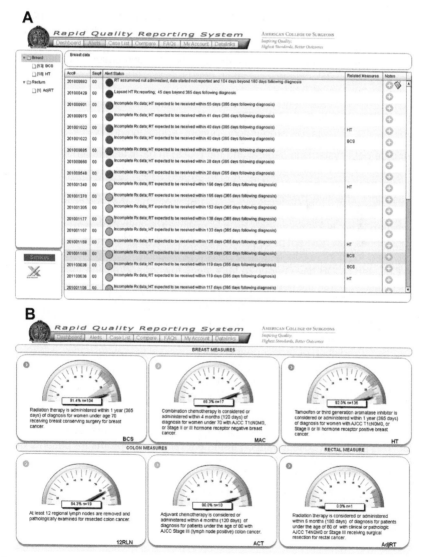

Fig. 2. RQRS screenshots. (*A*) Alerts screen indicating patients who have yet to receive recommended therapy. (*B*) Dashboards indicating year-to-date compliance rates.

Oncology Clinical Scholar-in-Residence program with the specific aim of training health services researchers interested in oncology. This unique two-year fellowship provides surgical residents with the opportunity to work at the American College of Surgeons on projects examining health care quality, health policy, and outcomes. As part of the fellowship, residents earn a Masters degree in health services research. So far, the program has been extremely successful, with almost 100 articles published as a result of the work of clinical scholars.

The NCDB also launched its Participant User File (PUF) initiative, whereby Health Insurance Portability and Accountability Act (HIPAA) compliant, de-identified patient level data are provided to investigators at CoC-approved cancer programs. The purpose of the PUF initiative is to provide qualified investigators with a data resource than can be used for analyses that promote review and advancement of the quality of care delivered to patients with cancer. To date, investigators from seven alpha test sites have participated in this program, producing publications examining everything from patterns of care to outcomes for several different cancers. The beta testing phase of the PUF program is currently underway, with anticipated distribution of about 40 analytic data files.

FUTURE WORK OF THE CoC AND NCDB

Although significant advancements have been made in the last decade to enhance cancer care data systems in general and the NCDB in particular, much work remains to be done. Registry data currently do not incorporate patient-reported outcomes, which is a necessary component for a rounded assessment of health care quality. Also, as more effective therapies are discovered, cancer is increasingly a chronic disease with the attendant difficulties of good, long-term follow-up in a fragmented care system. This is compounded by the reality of hospital infrastructure that, in many instances, has not kept pace with the globalization and information age changes that have led to an increasingly mobile patient population.

The CoC and NCDB have begun to take steps toward addressing these issues via several initiatives. First, the new cancer program standards for CoC-accreditation that go into effect in 2012 are all focused on increasing patient-centered care. CoC hospitals will be required to provide the following services: risk assessment and genetic counseling; palliative care services; a patient navigation process, in which patients and caregivers are given individualized assistance to overcome barriers to care; and survivorship care plans.[26] Next, the NCDB is actively developing an online tool or program that will use submitted patient data to produce a summary of the patient's disease and treatment up to that point and can thus serve as the template for generating a survivorship care plan. Finally, in a study using RQRS as the case finding and data entry platform, the NCDB in collaboration with the NCI and American Cancer Society will examine patient-reported outcomes for patients with breast and colorectal cancer. This study will collect data on treatment-related symptoms for patients diagnosed with these tumors at 16 cancer centers participating in the NCI Community Cancer Center Program. This study should provide proof of concept for this next frontier in the use of registry data to affect quality.

REFERENCES

1. Soni A. Top 10 most costly conditions among men and women, 2008: estimates for the U.S. civilian noninstitutionalized adult population, age 18 and older. Statistical brief 331. Rockville (MD): Agency for Healthcare Research and Quality. Available

at: http://www.meps.ahrq.gov/mepsweb/data_files/publications/st331/stat331.pdf. Accessed October 30, 2011.

2. Meropol NJ, Schulman KA. Cost of cancer care: issues and implications. J Clin Oncol 2007;25:180–6.

3. Hewitt M, Simone JV, editors. Institute of Medicine. Ensuring quality cancer care. Washington, DC: National Academy Press; 1999.

4. Hewitt M, Simone JV, editors. Institute of Medicine. Enhancing data systems to improve the quality of cancer care. Washington, DC: National Academy Press; 2000.

5. National Program of Cancer Registries (NPCR). Available at: http://www.cdc.gov/cancer/npcr/about.htm. Accessed October 30, 2011.

6. Surveillance epidemiology and end results. Available at: http://seer.cancer.gov/about/overview.html. Accessed October 30, 2011.

7. Winchester DP, Stewart AK, Bura C, et al. The National Cancer Data Base: a clinical surveillance and quality improvement tool. J Surg Oncol 2004;85(1):1–3.

8. Bilimoria KY, Bentrem DJ, Stewart AK, et al. Comparison of Commission on Cancer-approved and -nonapproved hospitals in the United States. J Clin Oncol 2009;27:4177–81.

9. Bilimoria KY, Stewart AK, Winchester DP, et al. The National Cancer Data Base: a powerful initiative to improve cancer care in the United States. Ann Surg Oncol 2008;15(3):683–90.

10. Facility Oncology Registry Data Standards. Commission on Cancer, CoC/American College of Surgeons; 2011.

11. North American Association of Central Cancer Registries (NAACCR). Standards for cancer registries, volume II. Available at: http://www.naaccr.org/LinkClick.aspx?fileticket=3-5u5N3X71k%3d&tabid=133&mid=473. Accessed November 4, 2011.

12. Donabedian A. Evaluating the quality of medical care. Milbank Mem Fund Q 1965;44(Suppl):166–206.

13. Solberg LI, Mosser G, McDonald S. The three faces of performance measurement: improvement, accountability, and research. Jt Comm J Qual Improv 1997;23:135–47.

14. Nelson EC, Splaine ME, Batalden PB, et al. Building measurement and data collection into medical practice. Ann Intern Med 1998;128:460–6.

15. National Quality Forum. A national framework for healthcare quality measurement and reporting. Available at: http://www.qualityforum.org/Publications/2002/07/A_National_Framework_for_He0althcare_Quality_Measurement_and_Reporting.aspx. Accessed November 4, 2011.

16. Desch CE, McNiff KK, Schneider EC, et al. American Society of Clinical Oncology/National Comprehensive Cancer Network Quality Measures. J Clin Oncol 2008; 26(21):3631–7.

17. Collaborative Stage Data Collection System (CS). Available at: http://www.cancerstaging.org/cstage/about.html. Accessed November 4, 2011.

18. Malin JL, Kahn KL, Adams J, et al. Validity of cancer registry data for measuring the quality of breast cancer care. J Natl Cancer Inst 2002;94(11):835–44.

19. German RR, Wike JM, Bauer KR, et al, Patterns of Care Study Group. Quality of cancer registry data: findings from CDC-NPCR's Breast and Prostate Cancer Data Quality and Patterns of Care Study. J Registry Manag 2011; 38(2):75–86.

20. Warren JL, Klabunde CN, Schrag D, et al. Overview of the SEER-Medicare data: content, research applications, and generalizability to the United States elderly population. Med Care 2002;40(Suppl 8):IV3–18.

21. American College of Surgeons, Cancer Programs. Cancer Program Practice Profile Reports (CP3R). Available at: http://www.facs.org/cancer/ncdb/cp3r. html. Accessed November 7, 2011.
22. Pappas DP, Garbus JE, Feuerman M, et al. Improving uniformity of care for colorectal cancers through National Quality Forum quality indicators at a commission on cancer-accredited community based teaching hospital. Surg Oncol Clin N Am 2011;20(3):587–96.
23. Lodrigues W, Dumas J, Rao M, et al. Compliance with the commission on cancer quality of breast cancer care measures: self-evaluation advised. Breast J 2011; 17(2):167–71.
24. American College of Surgeons, Cancer Programs. Rapid Quality Reporting System (RQRS). Available at: http://www.facs.org/cancer/ncdb/rqrs.html. Accessed November 7, 2011.
25. Lipscomb J, Gillespie TW. State-level cancer quality assessment and research: building and sustaining the data infrastructure. Cancer J 2011;17(4):246–56.
26. Cancer Program Standards 2012: Ensuring Patient-Centered Care. Commission on Cancer, 2011.

Variation in Mortality After High-Risk Cancer Surgery
Failure to Rescue

Amir A. Ghaferi, MD, MS, Justin B. Dimick, MD, MPH*

KEYWORDS

- Cancer surgery • Mortality rate • Failure to rescue • Postoperative complication

KEY POINTS

- Variations in hospital mortality rates with oncologic resections vary widely.
- Failure to rescue seems to play an important role in these differences.
- Hospital resources and the attitudes and behaviors among caregivers in inpatient wards and ICUs may affect the ability to effectively rescue patients from major surgical complications.

Thousands of Americans die every year undergoing elective cancer surgery. A much larger number experience serious complications often associated with residual disability or reduced longevity. Wide variations in mortality rates across both hospitals and surgeons suggest that the safety of cancer surgery could be improved substantially, but efforts to improve quality are currently limited by a lack of understanding about exactly why some hospitals have poorer outcomes than others.

Mechanisms underlying variations in hospital mortality rates are not well understood. Elucidating the clinical mechanisms underlying these variations is important to develop more effective strategies for quality improvement. That hospitals with high mortality rates simply have higher complication rates is a common notion. Indeed, many organizations, including the Centers for Medicare and Medicaid Services (CMS), focus their quality improvement efforts on reducing complications. However, there is a growing body of evidence suggesting that complications and mortality are not related, that is, hospitals with high rates of complications do not necessarily have high rates of mortality. Thus, there must be other explanations for the existing hospital variations in mortality rates. One such explanation may be that hospitals with high mortality rates may not be proficient at recognizing and managing serious complications once they occur, a phenomenon known as failure to rescue.[1,2]

Center for Healthcare Outcomes and Policy (CHOP), Department of Surgery, University of Michigan, 2800 Plymouth Road, Building 520, Room 3144, Ann Arbor, MI 48109, USA
* Corresponding author.
E-mail address: jdimick@med.umich.edu

Surg Oncol Clin N Am 21 (2012) 389–395
doi:10.1016/j.soc.2012.03.006
1055-3207/12/$ – see front matter © 2012 Elsevier Inc. All rights reserved.
surgonc.theclinics.com

Answers to such questions have obvious implications for the types of quality improvements that are likely to be effective in cancer surgery. Evidence that excess mortality is attributable primarily to the development of complications would imply the need for interventions aimed at processes related to perioperative care. Variation in failure to rescue rates would instead suggest the need to focus on processes related to the recognition and management of major postoperative complications.

UNDERSTANDING WIDE VARIATIONS IN SURGICAL MORTALITY

More than 100,000 patients undergo major cancer resections each year in the United States. Many of these procedures are complex and associated with high rates of mortality.[3] Previous research suggests that morbidity and mortality rates are strongly influenced by the hospital and by the surgeon who performs the oncologic operation. Although robust, risk-adjusted provider-specific data on performance are generally lacking for cancer surgery, there is little doubt that patient outcomes vary as a function of hospital volume, surgeon volume, and surgical specialty training.[4–9] Variations in provider performance can have a major cumulative effect on patient prognosis. For example, one analysis estimated that patients undergoing surgery for colon, lung, or pancreatic cancer lose between 6 and 18 months of life expectancy in being treated at low-volume hospitals.[10]

Such data suggest opportunities for improving the quality of cancer surgery in the United States. This could occur by 2 alternative mechanisms: Selective referral, cancer surgery patients could be directed to hospitals (or surgeons) likely to get the best results; Quality improvement, aimed at making cancer surgery safer and more effective in the settings in which it is currently being performed. This article focuses on the latter.

Increased postoperative complication rates are generally attributed to increased mortality. Several studies have found that higher mortality rates at poorly performing hospitals are due to more frequent complications.[11,12] However, there is a growing body of evidence that complication incidence and mortality do not share a causal pathway at the hospital level.[8,9,13] For example, a retrospective study of coronary artery bypass grafting using national hospital discharge data found that after adjusting for patient severity, there were no correlations between hospital complication rates and hospital mortality rates.[14] Furthermore, other investigators have demonstrated through advanced statistical methods that patient characteristics (ie, age, gender, race, and comorbidities) account for postoperative complications and hospital characteristics (ie, number of beds, percentage of board certified surgeons and anesthesiologists, and nurse to bed ratios) account more for hospital mortality.[15] Historically, operative mortality rates and complication rates have been used as quality indicators for the hospital and surgeon; however, there are clearly some pitfalls to using these imprecise measures. Therefore, Silber and colleagues[1] introduced a new measure called failure to rescue. The original description of failure to rescue used a low-mortality operation, open cholecystectomy. Even so, there was a significant association between failure to rescue and variations in mortality rates for open cholecystectomy. More importantly, the investigators found that failure to rescue was associated more with hospital characteristics than patient factors, which provided some insight into the understanding of variations in mortality rates across hospitals.

RECENT ADVANCES IN KNOWLEDGE

Although previous studies could be criticized by their reliance on administrative data (and their limitations regarding risk adjustment and identification of complications), their main findings were subsequently confirmed by the authors' study published last year in the *New England Journal of Medicine*.[2] Based on detailed clinical data from American College of Surgeons National Surgical Quality Improvement Program , the authors' ranked 186 participating hospitals based on their overall risk-adjusted mortality rates and grouped them into quintiles. As seen in **Fig. 2**, hospitals with high mortality rates and those low mortality rates had virtually identical rates of complications and those of major complications. Instead, hospitals with low mortality rates were distinguished by how well they minimized mortality once a complication had occurred, that is, how well they rescued patients (**Fig. 1**).

These findings show the importance of timely recognition and effective management of postoperative complications and have obvious implications for the types of strategies likely to reduce surgical mortality.

UNDERSTANDING FAILURE TO RESCUE

Understanding what leads to increased rates of failure to rescue has yet to be determined. Although recent studies have demonstrated the important association between variations in hospital mortality rates and failure to rescue,[2,16] there is a scant body of evidence evaluating hospital characteristics associated with failure to rescue.[17,18] There is some empiric evidence suggesting several candidate factors. Multiple hospital-level resources could provide reasonable insight into failure-to-rescue, such as nurse to patient ratios, hospital size, presence of certified intensivists, availability of cardiac catheterization laboratories, and high-technology equipment. For example, Silber and colleagues[17] recently demonstrated the importance of hospital-teaching intensity in survival after general, vascular, and orthopedic surgery. Patients undergoing surgery at hospitals with high teaching intensity had a 15% lower odds of death. However, although complication rates did not vary widely, the rates of failure to rescue were very important in explaining the differences in outcomes at teaching hospitals. The successful rescue of a patient who develops a postoperative complication relies heavily on hospital systems and teamwork. The sequence of events following the development

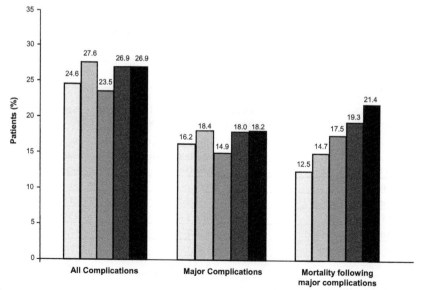

Fig. 1. Complications and mortality following major complications for hospital quintiles of risk-adjusted mortality.

of a major complication, such as a pulmonary embolism, can be very different depending on established hospital pathways or communication systems. For example, a nurse's role in identification of a hypoxic patient with dyspnea is an integral sentinel event in the management of this complication. The nurse must then communicate his/her findings to the surgeon effectively and ensure that timely intervention or reassessment occurs. Further, the availability of adjunctive radiologic studies and timely availability and administration of intravenous heparin are some examples of hospital resources and health care team systems that can make the difference between a positive or negative outcome. The importance of such factors has been established in the literature. For example, Pronovost and colleagues[19] identified approximately a 3-fold decrease in postoperative mortality rates of patients with abdominal aortic aneurysm repairs with daily rounds by the physicians in intensive care unit. Furthermore, Friese and colleagues[20] found a 37% increased odds of death for patients undergoing oncologic surgery in hospitals with poor nursing environments. These are just a few examples of possible hospital level factors that may influence the ability of hospitals to rescue patients from major complications.

In addition, although not directly examining failure to rescue, there have been several studies examining hospital attributes associated with surgical mortality.[1,19,21,22] For example, there is a large body of work supporting the notion that favorable nursing environments can help reducing the rates of surgical mortality.[20,23–27] In a study of hospitals in Pennsylvania, Aiken and colleagues[25] found that each additional patient per nurse was associated with a 7% increase in the likelihood of dying within 30 days of surgery. The authors' recent studies build on this existing work by demonstrating that these associations with mortality are likely mediated through an impact on the rates of failure to rescue.

Teaching status, nurse staffing, and hospital technology have been identified as the 3 factors most highly associated with failure to rescue (**Table 1**). Clinically, it is intuitive that these hospital attributes would provide an environment conducive to timely recognition and management of major complications. For example, first, a nurse who has fewer patients to care for may quickly identify a postoperative patient with acute hypoxia. Next, having house staff present 24 hours a day, 7 days a week would allow for rapid communication of this finding to a physician who could then initiate the appropriate evaluation. Finally, particular hospital systems (ie, electronic medication ordering and availability of advanced radiographic capabilities) may increase the

Table 1
Effect of each hospital characteristic on the odds of failure to rescue at a hospital with very high mortality rate compared with a hospital with a very low mortality rate

Hospital Characteristic	Odds Ratio [95% CI] Adjusted for Hospital Characteristic[a]	Proportion of Failure to Rescue Explained (%)
All characteristics	6.6 [3.7–11.9]	36.0
High hospital technology	7.7 [4.3–13.6]	24.0
Teaching hospital	7.8 [4.5–13.6]	23.0
Increased nurse to patient ratio	8.3 [4.7–14.6]	17.0
Hospital size >200 beds	8.9 [5.1–15.3]	11.0
Average daily census >50% capacity	9.6 [5.6–16.4]	3.0

Abbreviation: CI, confidence interval.
  [a] Odds ratio of failure to rescue in patients at hospitals with very high mortality rate compared to those with very low mortality rate.

likelihood of this patient receiving the appropriate diagnosis or intervention.[28,29] Although these are plausible clinical explanations for the observed associations in our study, a causal link cannot be established using these data (see **Table 1**).

FUTURE DIRECTIONS

The hospital attributes mentioned previously may simply be proxy measures for effective processes of care or hospital cultures conducive to the early recognition and effective management of complications. Most perioperative deaths are the culmination of a cascade of discrete clinical events (**Fig. 2**). Patients doing well at first suffer an initial or seminal complication followed by escalation of care, additional domino complications, and ultimately death. This chain of events can be influenced or interrupted by timely recognition and effective action taking along the way. In turn, recognition and action are influenced by both the availability of specific types of hospital resources and by the behaviors and attitudes among caregivers in inpatient wards and ICUs where postoperative patients receive their care. Future work should attempt to elucidate the details of care that lead to the effective rescue of patients from surgical complications. For example, increasing adherence to evidence-based processes of care, such as the successful Surviving Sepsis Campaign, may improve rescue rates at poorly performing hospitals.[30] Timely implementation of the Surviving Sepsis guidelines has proven to reduce mortality rates and ICU length of stay by up to 30%.[31] Although some may argue that the Surviving Sepsis Campaign was successful solely based on the implementation of a standardized protocol, one cannot ignore the importance of the Campaign's creation of an atmosphere with increased awareness of these life-saving evidence-based measures. Although discrete processes of care account for some of the variation in rescue rates, hospital culture also definitely plays a role. Previous work has described organizational factors, such as safety climate and morale; work environment factors, such as staffing levels; and team factors, such as teamwork and supervision, as influential in clinical practice.[32] However, measuring

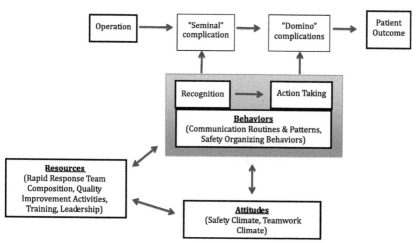

Fig. 2. Conceptual model outlining the interaction between hospital resources, behaviors, and attitudes in the early recognition and effective management of major postoperative complications.

hospital cultures or climates can be difficult. Quantitative surveys, such as the Safety Attitudes Questionnaire, have been implemented to learn more about the framework of systems in which surgical care is delivered.[33,34] Yet, to fully understand the factors that enable a hospital to have very low rates of failure to rescue, a mixed methods approach with site visits would allow us to gain insights into the effective and ineffective strategies of postoperative care. Focus groups and in-depth interviews could target key informants involved in the care of surgical patients with complications, including members of the inpatient ward, intensive care unit, and rapid response teams. A better understanding of these microsystems within hospitals could provide important actionable insights into how hospitals can improve their ability to rescue patients (see **Fig. 2**).

REFERENCES

1. Silber JH, Williams SV, Krakauer H, et al. Hospital and patient characteristics associated with death after surgery. A study of adverse occurrence and failure to rescue. Med Care 1992;30:615–29.
2. Ghaferi AA, Birkmeyer JD, Dimick JB. Variation in hospital mortality associated with inpatient surgery. N Engl J Med 2009;361:1368–75.
3. Finks JF, Osborne NH, Birkmeyer JD. Trends in hospital volume and operative mortality for high-risk surgery. N Engl J Med 2011;364:2128–37.
4. Bianco FJ Jr, Riedel ER, Begg CB, et al. Variations among high volume surgeons in the rate of complications after radical prostatectomy: further evidence that technique matters. J Urol 2005;173:2099–103.
5. Birkmeyer JD, Siewers AE, Finlayson EV, et al. Hospital volume and surgical mortality in the United States. N Engl J Med 2002;346:1128–37.
6. Birkmeyer JD, Stukel TA, Siewers AE, et al. Surgeon volume and operative mortality in the United States. N Engl J Med 2003;349:2117–27.
7. Finlayson EV, Goodney PP, Birkmeyer JD. Hospital volume and operative mortality in cancer surgery: a national study. Arch Surg 2003;138:721–5 [discussion: 6].
8. Dudley RA, Johansen KL, Brand R, et al. Selective referral to high-volume hospitals: estimating potentially avoidable deaths. JAMA 2000;283:1159–66.
9. Halm EA, Lee C, Chassin MR. Is volume related to outcome in health care? A systematic review and methodologic critique of the literature. Ann Intern Med 2002;137:511–20.
10. Finlayson EV, Birkmeyer JD. Effects of hospital volume on life expectancy after selected cancer operations in older adults: a decision analysis. J Am Coll Surg 2003;196:410–7.
11. Khuri SF, Henderson WG, DePalma RG, et al. Determinants of long-term survival after major surgery and the adverse effect of postoperative complications. Ann Surg 2005;242:326–41 [discussion: 41–3].
12. Silber JH, Rosenbaum PR, Trudeau ME, et al. Changes in prognosis after the first postoperative complication. Med Care 2005;43:122–31.
13. Houghton A. Variation in outcome of surgical procedures. Br J Surg 1994;81:653–60.
14. Silber JH, Rosenbaum PR, Schwartz JS, et al. Evaluation of the complication rate as a measure of quality of care in coronary artery bypass graft surgery. JAMA 1995;274:317–23.
15. Silber JH, Rosenbaum PR, Ross RN. Comparing the contributions of groups of predictors: which outcomes vary with hospital rather than patient characteristics? J Am Stat Assoc 1995;90:7–18.

16. Ghaferi AA, Birkmeyer JD, Dimick JB. Complications, failure to rescue, and mortality with major inpatient surgery in medicare patients. Ann Surg 2009;250: 1029–34.
17. Silber JH, Rosenbaum PR, Romano PS, et al. Hospital teaching intensity, patient race, and surgical outcomes. Arch Surg 2009;144:113–20 [discussion: 21].
18. Silber JH, Romano PS, Rosen AK, et al. Failure-to-rescue: comparing definitions to measure quality of care. Med Care 2007;45:918–25.
19. Pronovost PJ, Jenckes MW, Dorman T, et al. Organizational characteristics of intensive care units related to outcomes of abdominal aortic surgery. JAMA 1999;281:1310–7.
20. Friese CR, Lake ET, Aiken LH, et al. Hospital nurse practice environments and outcomes for surgical oncology patients. Health Serv Res 2008;43:1145–63.
21. Rosenthal GE, Harper DL, Quinn LM, et al. Severity-adjusted mortality and length of stay in teaching and nonteaching hospitals. Results of a regional study. JAMA 1997;278:485–90.
22. Pronovost PJ, Angus DC, Dorman T, et al. Physician staffing patterns and clinical outcomes in critically ill patients: a systematic review. JAMA 2002;288:2151–62.
23. Aiken LH, Clarke SP, Cheung RB, et al. Educational levels of hospital nurses and surgical patient mortality. JAMA 2003;290:1617–23.
24. Aiken LH, Clarke SP, Silber JH, et al. Hospital nurse staffing, education, and patient mortality. LDI Issue Brief 2003;9:1–4.
25. Aiken LH, Clarke SP, Sloane DM, et al. Hospital nurse staffing and patient mortality, nurse burnout, and job dissatisfaction. JAMA 2002;288:1987–93.
26. Friese CR. Nurse practice environments and outcomes: implications for oncology nursing. Oncol Nurs Forum 2005;32:765–72.
27. Sasichay-Akkadechanunt T, Scalzi CC, Jawad AF. The relationship between nurse staffing and patient outcomes. J Nurs Adm 2003;33:478–85.
28. Pickering BW, Hurley K, Marsh B. Identification of patient information corruption in the intensive care unit: using a scoring tool to direct quality improvements in handover. Crit Care Med 2009;37:2905–12.
29. Chen J, Krumholz HM, Wang Y, et al. Differences in patient survival after acute myocardial infarction by hospital capability of performing percutaneous coronary intervention: implications for regionalization. Arch Intern Med 2010;170:433–9.
30. Dellinger RP, Levy MM, Carlet JM, et al. Surviving Sepsis Campaign: international guidelines for management of severe sepsis and septic shock: 2008. Crit Care Med 2008;36:296–327.
31. Zambon M, Ceola M, Almeida-de-Castro R, et al. Implementation of the Surviving Sepsis Campaign guidelines for severe sepsis and septic shock: we could go faster. J Crit Care 2008;23:455–60.
32. Vincent C, Taylor-Adams S, Stanhope N. Framework for analysing risk and safety in clinical medicine. BMJ 1998;316:1154–7.
33. Pronovost PJ, Berenholtz SM, Goeschel C, et al. Improving patient safety in intensive care units in Michigan. J Crit Care 2008;23:207–21.
34. Sexton JB, Helmreich RL, Neilands TB, et al. The Safety Attitudes Questionnaire: psychometric properties, benchmarking data, and emerging research. BMC Health Serv Res 2006;6:44.

Unexpected Readmissions After Major Cancer Surgery

An Evaluation of Readmissions as a Quality-of-Care Indicator

Matthew M. Rochefort, MD[a], James S. Tomlinson, MD, PhD[b,c],*

KEYWORDS

- Surgery • Readmission • Rehospitalization • Oncology • Quality care

KEY POINTS

- Readmission rates following major cancer surgery are between 16% to 25% at 30 days and 53% to 66% at 1 year.
- Review of the literature revealed several risk factors predictive of readmissions, such as age, comorbidities, and hospital length of stay.
- Future readmission studies are needed to evaluate the global processes of surgical care and their impact on readmission rates. The authors provide a conceptual framework for conduction of these studies in a prospective manner.
- The proposed congressional plan to use readmission rates to assess hospital performance and determine reimbursement should be pursued with extreme caution, pending further investigation.

A major oncologic operation carries a significant level of stress on the physical and mental well-being of a patient. This stress can be greatly exacerbated by an unexpected hospital readmission, with potential impact on quality of life from a physiologic, psychologic, social, and economic standpoint.[1] Beyond the obvious effects on the patient and the possibility of delaying further adjuvant treatments, unexpected readmissions have a significant impact on hospital resources and are a considerable

[a] Department of Surgery, David Geffen School of Medicine at UCLA, 10833 Le Conte Avenue, Room 54-140 CHS, Box 9511782, Los Angeles, CA 90095-1782, USA; [b] Department of Surgery, University of California, Los Angeles, David Geffen School of Medicine at UCLA, 10833 Le Conte Avenue, Room 54-140 CHS, Box 9511782, Los Angeles, CA 90095-1782, USA; [c] Surgical Oncology, Greater Los Angeles VA Medical Center, 11301 Wilshire Boulevard, Los Angeles, CA 90073, USA
* Corresponding author. Department of Surgery, University of California, Los Angeles, David Geffen School of Medicine at UCLA, 10833 Le Conte Avenue, Room 54-140 CHS, Box 9511782, Los Angeles, CA 90095-1782.
E-mail address: jtomlinson@mednet.ucla.edu

Surg Oncol Clin N Am 21 (2012) 397–405
doi:10.1016/j.soc.2012.03.004
1055-3207/12/$ – see front matter Published by Elsevier Inc.

surgonc.theclinics.com

source of the continuing rise in the cost of health care in the United States. A 2009 *New England Journal of Medicine* article reported that 20% of all Medicare patients are readmitted to the hospital within the first 30 days after discharge, resulting in an annual cost of over 17 billion dollars.[2] As national efforts continue to curb the cost of health care, hospital readmission rates have recently been brought to the forefront of public and congressional policymakers' attention. In 2007, the Medicare Payment Advisory Commission proposed the use of readmission rates as a quality performance measure.[3] Subsequently, in 2009, the Center for Medicare and Medicaid Services began requiring the reporting of 30-day hospital readmission rates for three of the most common admitting diagnoses: heart failure, pneumonia, and acute myocardial infarction.[4] It can only be assumed that, in the future, postoperative hospital readmissions will also fall under this umbrella of mandatory reporting and evaluation as a quality performance measure of inpatient surgical care.

Given the aforementioned interest in readmissions as an indicator of quality and the potential to adjust payment for readmissions, surgeons should take action to further develop and perfect the study of postoperative readmissions and evaluate the validity of using readmissions as a measure of quality. The first area of investigation should be to determine a universally accepted postoperative length of time for which an unexpected readmission is linked or related to the "quality" of the care delivered during the surgical admission. Most surgeons continue to fall back on 30-day morbidity and mortality as the time frame to be judged because it is generally assumed that the more time elapsed between discharge and readmission the less likely it is that the prior hospitalization played a significant role.[5] This is significantly shorter than the 90-day global period that Medicare has developed. The payment for a surgical procedure includes a standard package of preoperative, intraoperative, and postoperative services. The preoperative period included in the global fee for major surgery is 1 day and the postoperative period for major surgery is 90 days.[6] Thus, it seems that Medicare has defined 90 days as an appropriate length of time to hold the surgical care team accountable. However, this time frame for major oncologic operations should be scrutinized for validity before it is accepted. Considering that oncology patients are generally older with more comorbidities, unexpected and unpreventable postoperative hospital admissions may be higher at baseline compared with an operation for a benign condition.

Research into unexpected hospital readmissions has sought to define characteristics of and risk factors for those readmissions. They can essentially be broken down into four groups: preoperative risk factors (age, comorbidities, disease extent, cancer stage), initial hospitalization risk factors (length of operation, length of stay, perioperative complications), discharge disposition status (home alone, home with family, home with home health, rehabilitation facility, nursing home), and, finally, the reasons for readmission (operative complication, pneumonia, dehydration, bleeding). However, many of the currently available papers are lacking the ability to demonstrate a causal association between substandard inpatient care and early readmission, which would be the cornerstone of using readmission as a quality-care indicator.[5]

Outcomes and readmission data for most complex oncologic operations are generated from retrospective case series reviews of large, single institutions with a high volume of the specific operation being studied. As these institutions continue to develop broader geographic catchment areas, the ability for them to accurately record the absolute number of patient readmissions is decreasing. Patients are often willing to travel great distances, and across state lines, to have an operation at a high-volume center; however, often present to the closest available emergency room when postdischarge problems arise.[7] Therefore, the data from single-institution series often underestimate the actual readmission rate. Moreover, regionalization of major abdominal operations has been promoted given the positive volume–outcome relationship demonstrated in many complex oncologic procedures.[8] High-volume centers have demonstrated decreased operative time and hospital length of stay as evidence of improved quality of care.[7] Interestingly, as hospital length of stay has decreased it was speculated that the number of hospital readmissions due to conditions and complications that would have manifested during a longer initial hospitalization would be on the rise. This is not borne out by the data; in fact, an increase in initial hospital length of stay is commonly reported as an independent risk factor for future readmissions.[9,10]

Given the inaccuracy of hospital readmission rates from single-institution reports, recent effort has been put forth to extract population-level data from administrative data sets, including the Medicare fee-for-service database linked to state or national cancer registries (eg, the Surveillance, Epidemiology and End Results [SEER] registry). This type of linked data set provides accurate readmission data regarding dates, duration, and hospital of readmission. Linking this data with cancer registry data allows tumor-specific data (eg, American Joint Committee on Cancer stage and pathology) to be added and allows for proper stratification and comparison of outcomes.

One of the initial papers utilizing one of these large administrative data sets linked to a statewide cancer registry database was by Yermilov and colleagues.[7] They performed a population-based study for all patients in California undergoing a pancreaticoduodenectomy for adenocarcinoma between 1994 and 2003, which resulted in a patient cohort of 2023 patients. They demonstrated a 59% readmission rate in the first year, with 47% of those patients being readmitted to a hospital other then the one at which they had their operation. Advanced age, higher Charlson Comorbidity Index (CCI), higher T-stage, and longer initial hospitalization were all positive predictors of readmission. They also sought to bring attention to the causes of readmission, such as dehydration and electrolyte abnormalities, which they propose may have been prevented with the implementation of additional processes, such as patient education, home health services, and improved communication with primary care providers.

Administrative databases also attempt to collect data on comorbidities that are important to help risk adjust readmission data. The CCI, referred to in many of the following studies of surgical readmissions, is a weighted scale developed by epidemiologist Mary Charlson in 1987. It assigns a value to a patient's overall comorbidities in an attempt to assess risk for 1-year mortality.[11] It involves heart disease, vascular disease, pulmonary disease, diabetes, renal disease, liver disease, malignancy, and AIDS as potentially weighted conditions.[11] Charlson and colleagues[12] also combined an age-adjusted CCI with their standard comorbidity index to assess the additional mortality risk of patients greater than 40 years old. Articles researching outcomes in patients who have cancer occasionally use a modified CCI that removes malignancy as a weighted condition because this is assumed to be present in all the patients.[7] The CCI is an important tool in the preoperative risk assessment of a patient to determine what unmodifiable patient-level factors may contribute to risk for surgical complication and readmission.

In addition to the Yermilov and colleagues[7] study, the University of California Los Angeles, under the direction of Clifford Ko, has compiled data (Clifford Ko, unpublished, 2011) on early readmission rates (defined as within 30 days following surgical treatment of lung and gastrointestinal [GI] cancers) between 1994 and 2004. Preliminary results demonstrate that for patients undergoing surgical resection for stomach cancer (subsample size 12,769), the 30-day readmission rate is 25.6%, and the 1-year readmission rate approaches 66%. Similar to the Yermilov findings, positive predictors for readmission included increasing the CCI score, any hospitalization in the year before the operation, distant disease at the time of the operation, and increased length of stay following their surgery. Patients that were discharged to home were less likely to need a readmission within 30 days then those discharged elsewhere. The most common reason sited for readmission was a surgical complication accounting for 41% of readmissions. Surgical complications were followed by hypovolemia, pulmonary dysfunction, and nutrition, collectively accounting for another 47% of readmissions.

In 2010, Greenblatt and colleagues[13] published a population-based study using the SEER linked-Medicare database for all patients undergoing colectomy for colon cancer from 1992 to 2002. This study included 42,348 patients discharged after colectomy and demonstrated an 11% readmission rate within 30 days, with 13.2% of patients being readmitted to a hospital other than the one they initially had their surgery. The following factors were found to be predicative of readmission: male gender; hospitalization for any reason in the year before operation, comorbidities, nonelective surgery, prolonged hospital stay (>15 days), blood transfusion, ostomy creation, and discharge to a nursing home. Additionally they found a 1-year, stage-adjusted, survival advantage associated with patients who did not require a readmission, the magnitude of which was comparable to the difference in mortality between patients with stage I disease and those with stage III.

Reddy and colleagues[9] also used the SEER-Medicare–linked data from 1992 to 2003 for all patients undergoing pancreatic resection for adenocarcinoma (76% Whipple, 18% distal, 3% total, and 3% not otherwise specified). They found 1730 patients that met their criteria and demonstrated a 16% readmission rate at 30 days and 53% at 1 year. The reason for readmission was related to operative complications in 80% of patients readmitted within 30 days. Their definition of operative complication was quite broad and included abscesses, sepsis, hemorrhage, pancreatic fistula, GI bleed, urinary tract infection, pneumonia, respiratory failure, and venous thromboembolism or pulmonary embolism. Their analysis produced type of operation (distal pancreatectomy) and length of stay (>10 days) as predictive of early readmission, while age, race, sex, CCI, tumor stage, and node status were not found to statistically impact readmission rates. Interestingly, this study demonstrated that distal pancreatectomy had a higher rate of readmission than a pancreatic head resection. The investigators propose this may be partially due to higher rates of pancreatic leak and that distal pancreatectomies are less likely to be performed at high-volume centers.

These large population-based studies provide excellent baseline statistics for readmissions. They are able to effectively produce an accurate overall rate of readmission because they are capable of capturing all readmissions, even those to hospitals other than where the original operation was performed. The consensus between these studies is a readmission rate of 16% to 25% for major oncologic operations at 30 days and 53% to 66% at 1 year. They are also capable of providing global factors associated with readmission, such as increased length of hospitalization, any hospitalization in the year prior, and increased comorbidity index.

Medicare data and Medicare-linked databases are good sources of information on inpatient, outpatient, hospice, and home health claims for the elderly. However, the information may not be able to be generalized to the population at large because it is obtained only from those patients over 65 years of age. Medicare data are also limited in regard to lack of information on services not covered under the program and services reimbursed by third-party payers. Regarding cancer outcomes research, administrative data sets are often lacking because they do not contain information on the cancer stage or metastasis because these do not affect reimbursement. To overcome this limitation, as mentioned previously, administrative data sets are merged with a tumor registry such as SEER, National Cancer Data Base, or a statewide cancer registry. SEER data provide information on patient demographics as well as tumor grade, primary site, and extent of disease. Limitations within the SEER database include that the information obtained is not standardized and, whereas some tumors may be reported according to the TNM-staging criteria, others are reported more vaguely with descriptors such as "localized" or "distant." The very large sample size associated with administrative data sets also allows the potential to determine statistically significant differences ($P<.05$) even when the absolute difference is very small and possibly clinically insignificant.[14]

Another important limitation of administrative data sets includes a certain inherent level of bias because procedures that are reimbursed, such as operations or length of hospital stay, are likely to be more accurately recorded than subjective patient-level characteristics, such as the comorbidity status of a patient or complications. Although comorbidities tend to be undercoded, CCI data derived from administrative data perform well when compared with the index derived from medical record chart review.[14] Using claims data for risk assessment is also limited because there is no way to assess whether a specific diagnosis was present on admission or occurred during the hospitalization. In addition, each admission has a "principle diagnosis" code from *International Classification of Diseases, 9th Revision, Clinical Modification*. However, it also has up to 25 other diagnoses coded for that admission. One can imagine the confounding situation when the principle diagnosis for a readmission is recorded as "pancreas cancer" but the secondary diagnosis and true reason for early postoperative readmission is dehydration or biliary obstruction. This is a major limitation of analyses of administrative datasets in trying to assign true cause for readmission.

Although single-institution studies may not be able to produce the same accuracy of data regarding overall readmission rates, they are able, through chart review, to provide much more accurate accounts of reasons for readmissions and patient comorbidities at the time of admission. Furthermore, they are better prepared to assess hospital policies and health care processes, such as multidisciplinary discharge rounds, and the impact on rates and causes of readmission. The following three studies are single-institution studies designed to study their own rates of postoperative readmissions.

Beth Israel Deaconess Medical Center performed a review of all pancreatic resections performed at their facility between 2001 and 2009, resulting in 578 patients (371 Whipple, 187 distal, 11 total, and 9 other). They recorded a readmission rate of 19% in the first 30 days with only 2% of patients requiring readmission between 30 and 90 days. The only factors found related to risk of readmission were a small pancreatic duct, postoperative complications, and increased length of stay. Additionally, they demonstrated that patients discharged to home with home nursing required more readmissions then those sent home without nursing or those sent to a rehabilitation facility. The group also was able to evaluate the increase in cost associated with early readmission after pancreatic resection. They demonstrated a greater than 10,000 dollar cost associated with the readmission and, for those requiring readmission, their original hospitalization was, on average, 6000 dollars more expensive.[10]

Morris and colleagues[15] performed a retrospective case series analysis at the Hospital of the University of Pennsylvania of the administrative data for all discharges from their mixed surgical unit in 2009. They were able to show a 3% unexpected readmission rate within 30 days. They found that longer hospital length of stay as well as deep venous thrombosis or acute renal failures during the original hospitalization were associated with increased risk of readmission. The 30-day readmission rates were significantly below the national average of 10% to 20% and they proposed that this could be, in part, due to the lower average age of their patients or the use of daily multidisciplinary rounds, with social workers and discharge planners who carefully evaluate patient's needs and timely coordination of transitions in care.

In 2010, Stimson and colleagues[16] published a single-institution retrospective case series review of all radical cystectomies performed between 2001 and 2007 at Vanderbilt University Medical Center. They found a 26% readmission rate in the first 90 days and, of those, 19.7% were readmitted in the first 30 days. They showed gender, CCI, tumor stage, and any postoperative complication as independent predictors of 90-day readmission. The CCI was a significant risk factor because it demonstrated an odds ratio for readmission of 1.19 per unit increase in the composite score. For example, a patient with diabetes, previous myocardial infarct, and chronic pulmonary disease has a CCI score of 3 resulting in a 40% increased risk of being readmitted compared with a patient whose only comorbidity is diabetes (CCI score 1).

These single-institution studies were able to accurately record patient-level comorbidities and assess the impact of those comorbidities on rates of readmission. Additionally, they can more accurately assign the true "reason" or diagnosis associated with the readmission. This allows the hospital to assess their own policies and health care processes and make a rational determination of whether they have an impact on readmissions. Finally, single-institution studies allow for proposal and implementation of novel processes, derived from local-studies data, which may limit the number of future readmissions.

SUMMARY

Unexpected readmissions are a significant drain to hospital resources and are a contributing factor for the rising cost of health care in the United States. Outcomes, surgical complications, and readmission data for most complex oncologic operations are generated from retrospective case series of large single institutions with a high volume of the specific operation being studied. As patients travel greater distances to tertiary care centers for their complex operations, the ability of these retrospective studies to capture all of the readmissions decreases. In two large population-based studies, this is demonstrated by the difference in readmission rates to hospitals other than the one where the original operation was performed.[7,13] Greenblatt and colleagues[13] studied colectomy for colon cancer, which is commonly performed by general surgeons or colorectal surgeons in community hospitals. Yermilov and colleagues[7] studied pancreaticoduodenectomy, a complex operation that is being progressively performed only at high-volume centers. The difference in the readmission rates of patients to hospitals other than the one performing the operation was significant, with only 13% after colectomy and 47% after pancreaticoduodenectomy. Furthermore, studies that fail to account for the proportion of patients readmitted to a different hospital are ignoring the subset of patients that elect to be readmitted to a different hospital because of some perceived substandard care at the first hospital.

A readmission, although costly to the hospital and insurance payers, has an even more significant negative effect on the patient. It has been repeatedly demonstrated that patients requiring readmission after surgery have worse median survival than those not requiring readmission.[7,9,10,13] Many of these readmissions are potentially preventable. It has been demonstrated that patients surviving the initial insult of an early readmission have long-term survival similar to those not requiring an early readmission.[9] Thus, suggesting that the impact on median survival of these readmissions may be due to preventable or reversible acute problems arising early in the postoperative course.

Dehydration, venous thromboembolism, pulmonary embolism, pneumonia, gastritis, and GI bleed are commonly reported causes for hospital readmissions in the first 30 days postoperatively.[7,9,10,13,16] These causes represent a significant area for improvement because most, if not all, of these are potentially preventable causes of readmissions. For example, rates of readmission secondary to gastritis or GI bleed could be reduced with an intervention as simple and inexpensive as ensuring that all postoperative patients are discharged on acid suppressive therapy unless contraindicated. Further investigation is needed to review the specific causes for early readmission and develop steps that can be taken in the initial hospitalization and in the early postdischarge time frame to decrease preventable causes. Notably, most of the risk factors predictive of future readmissions are not modifiable, such as age, comorbidities, or a complication. However, they may serve as identifiers for patient preoperative and postoperative risk assessment. This assessment would reduce readmissions by allowing a more appropriate and candid patient-surgeon discussion about the risks, temper expectations, and perhaps dictate a higher level of vigilance in the postoperative period.

Extending the current readmission rate analysis beyond the 30-day window would provide a more accurate understanding of the cost, both in morbidity to patients and in costs to the institutions and insurers associated with major oncologic operations. This would also more properly align the research of readmissions with what Medicare has already deemed to be the appropriate window of 90-days. The obvious problem with a 90-day window when dealing with some aggressive cancers is progression of disease and the impact of adjuvant therapy. Most studies have supported the continuation of the 30-day window because most readmissions occur in the first 5 to 10 days and trend downward after that. Greenblatt and colleagues[7] and Yermilov and colleagues[13] show histograms showing the number of readmissions per postdischarge day. The graphs demonstrate that most readmissions occur in the first 2 weeks and then trail off significantly. However, these studies do not demonstrate a trend to zero and a significant number of patients continue to be readmitted in this later time frame.

Patients sometimes have unrealistic expectations of how quickly they will return to full functional status and, in very anxious patients, may cause them to request readmission prematurely.[1] This circumstance may be preventable with improved preoperative and discharge patient education and assessment of home-environment needs.[15] Postdischarge care is equally important. Patients with timely and appropriate postdischarge visits with their primary care provider may be less likely to require readmission. A dedicated study in this area, however, is not available. Readmissions may be a better indicator of the spectrum of both inpatient and postdischarge care rather than simply inpatient care.[5] Further investigation is necessary to understand the relative contributions of failures in discharge planning, insufficient outpatient resources, underuse of supportive palliative care programs, and progression of disease to the overall risk of hospital readmissions after major oncologic surgery.

The proposed plan of using readmission rates to assess hospital performance and of using them as a performance measure for reimbursement should be pursued with caution. Brown and colleagues[1] perhaps states this best in an editorial with a well-worded analogy. They ask the readers to consider three potential outcomes from peritonitis: the patient gets better, the patient develops an abscess, or the patient dies. Development of an abscess, although costly and unfortunate, is a profoundly better outcome than death. This benefit should not be looked on as a failure and it would

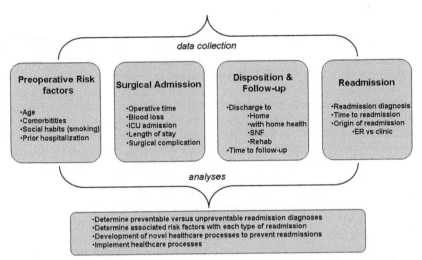

Fig. 1. Conceptual framework for institutional study of disease specific readmissions. ER, emergency room; SNF, skilled nursing facility.

generally be considered unfair to punish a hospital and withhold payment because of an event that is part of a natural course of a disease process. As such, surgical complications are inherent risks associated with complex oncologic surgeries and may not be preventable and do lead to early postoperative readmissions.

Large population-based data sets provide a comprehensive denominator for incidence, timing, and generalized reasons for readmission—the proverbial view from 30,000 feet. These studies are met, however, with several limitations that have been previously discussed. In the future, well-kept databases of detailed information at the individual hospital level will be necessary to assess a causal relationship between the specific hospital care delivered and the risk of readmission. Developing a framework for readmission data collection will be necessary for this research to progress. Given the review of the literature presented, the authors suggest the following four categories of readmission data be collected at the institutional level: (1) preoperative risk factors, (2) surgical admission data, (3) discharge disposition and follow up, and (4) readmission data (**Fig. 1**). Once this data is collected, it will be up to local experts to analyze it and determine if a readmission diagnosis is preventable or unpreventable. The factors from the four categories that are associated with potentially preventable readmissions should lead to development and implementation of novel processes aimed at decreasing readmissions.

REFERENCES

1. Brown RE, Qadan M, Martin RC 2nd, et al. The evolving importance of readmission data to the practicing surgeon. J Am Coll Surg 2010;211:558–60.
2. Jencks SF, Williams MV, Coleman EA. Rehospitalizations among patients in the Medicare fee-for-service program. N Engl J Med 2009;360:1418–28.
3. Medicare Payment Advisory Commission (U.S.). Report to the Congress: promoting greater efficiency in Medicare. Washington, DC: MedPAC; 2007.
4. Centers for Medicare & Medicaid Services. Fact sheet: quality measures for reporting in fiscal year 2009 for 2010 update. Baltimore (MD): Department of Health & Human Services; 2008.

5. Ashton CM, Wray NP. A conceptual framework for the study of early readmission as an indicator of quality of care. Soc Sci Med 1996;43:1533–41.
6. Medicare A/B Reference Manual. Chapter 22-Global Surgery and Related Services. Available at: https://www.novitas-solutions.com/refman/chapter-22.html. Accessed March 10, 2012.
7. Yermilov I, Bentrem D, Sekeris E, et al. Readmissions following pancreaticoduo-denectomy for pancreas cancer: a population-based appraisal. Ann Surg Oncol 2009;16:554–61.
8. Begg CB, Cramer LD, Hoskins WJ, et al. Impact of hospital volume on operative mortality for major cancer surgery. JAMA 1998;280:1747–51.
9. Reddy DM, Townsend CM Jr, Kuo YF, et al. Readmission after pancreatectomy for pancreatic cancer in medicare patients. J Gastrointest Surg 2009;13:1963–74 [discussion: 1974–5].
10. Kent TS, Sachs TE, Callery MP, et al. Readmission after major pancreatic resection: a necessary evil? J Am Coll Surg 2011;213(4):515–23. [Epub 2011 Aug 16].
11. Charlson ME, Pompei P, Ales KL, et al. A new method of classifying prognostic comorbidity in longitudinal studies: development and validation. J Chronic Dis 1987;40:373–83.
12. Charlson M, Szatrowski TP, Peterson J, et al. Validation of a combined comorbidity index. J Clin Epidemiol 1994;47:1245–51.
13. Greenblatt DY, Weber SM, O'Connor ES, et al. Readmission after colectomy for cancer predicts one-year mortality. Ann Surg 2010;251:659–69.
14. Nathan H, Pawlik TM. Limitations of claims and registry data in surgical oncology research. Ann Surg Oncol 2008;15:415–23.
15. Morris DS, Rohrbach J, Rogers M, et al. The surgical revolving door: risk factors for hospital readmission. J Surg Res 2011;170(2):297–301.
16. Stimson CJ, Chang SS, Barocas DA, et al. Early and late perioperative outcomes following radical cystectomy: 90-day readmissions, morbidity and mortality in a contemporary series. J Urol 2010;184:1296–300.

Importance of and Adherence to Lymph Node Staging Standards in Gastrointestinal Cancer

Ryan P. Merkow, MD[a,b,c], David J. Bentrem, MD, MS[d,*]

KEYWORDS

- Gastrointestinal cancer • Lymph nodes • Lymphadenectomy • Survival • Outcomes
- Quality improvement • Surgery

KEY POINTS

- Lymph node status is one of the most important predictors of survival in gastrointestinal cancer.
- The number of lymph nodes examined after surgical resection considerably affects staging accuracy, which is relevant for treatment decisions and when stratifying patients in clinical trials.
- For colon and rectal cancers, at least 12 lymph nodes should be examined after surgical resection; however, for other cancer sites and after neoadjuvant therapy, the precise number of nodes required is less clearly established.
- Current evidence suggests that there is lack of adequate lymph node examination across all gastrointestinal cancers in the United States.

In 2010, there were an estimated 1.5 million incident cases of cancer in the United States and nearly 600,000 deaths.[1] Approximately 17% of all new cases originated in the gastrointestinal (GI) tract but represented a quarter of all cancer-related deaths. Certain GI malignancies have an especially poor prognosis, particularly esophageal (5-year survival, 19%) and pancreatic (5-year survival, 6%) tumors.[1] The most common GI malignancy, colorectal cancer, represents nearly 10% of all diagnosed malignancies and cancer-related deaths in the United States.[1]

Given these statistics, it is imperative to identify strategies that improve the quality of cancer care in GI oncology. One of the most important predictors of survival is the presence of lymph node metastasis; however, the precise number of examined lymph nodes needed for accurate staging of each cancer site is variable and not always clearly

[a] Department of Surgery and Surgical Outcomes and Quality Improvement Center, Northwestern University Feinberg School of Medicine, Chicago, IL, USA; [b] Department of Surgery, University of Colorado, School of Medicine, Aurora, CO, USA; [c] Division of Research and Optimal Patient Care, American College of Surgeons, Chicago, IL, USA; [d] Division of Surgical Oncology, Department of Surgery, Northwestern University Feinberg School of Medicine, 676 North Saint Clair Street, Suite 650, Chicago, IL 60611, USA
* Corresponding author.
E-mail address: DBentrem@nmff.org

Surg Oncol Clin N Am 21 (2012) 407–416
doi:10.1016/j.soc.2012.03.010
1055-3207/12/$ – see front matter © 2012 Elsevier Inc. All rights reserved.
surgonc.theclinics.com

defined. Nevertheless, the number of lymph nodes examined after surgical resection considerably affects staging accuracy, which is relevant for treatment decisions and when stratifying patients in clinical trials. In addition, evidence suggests that the extent of lymphadenectomy could be a surrogate of other unmeasured factors, such as the quality of surgical technique, more thorough pathologic examination, or both.[2] Therefore, to address these issues, this article aims to explore current evidence and controversies with respect to lymph node staging standards in GI oncology.

HISTORY

The concept that lymph nodes may act as functional barriers and channels of cancer spread began to be accepted by the mid 1800s. Immediately after, William Halsted, an American-born surgeon, popularized the idea that cancer spreads in an orderly manner by way of lymphatic channels. Based on his own theory, Halsted[3] advocated radical mastectomy for treating women with breast cancer, an operation that removes the breast, underlying muscles, and all lymphatic tissues in the axilla. In this manner, Halsted believed that he was removing all locoregional diseases, particularly cancer cells harbored in axillary lymph nodes, which he postulated would decrease recurrence and ultimately improve survival.

Nevertheless, the role of lymph node sampling in the natural history of cancer continued to evolve. In contrast to the Halstedian theory, a new concept championed by Bernard Fisher and Blake Cady emerged. Fisher in particular believed that lymph node involvement was more an indicator of cancer biology than a step in the sequence toward distant metastases. He did not believe that variations in locoregional therapy were as important as addressing the systemic disease, and pushed for less radical surgical treatments.[4] Fisher went on to cofound the National Surgical Adjuvant Breast and Bowel project and conduct a series of landmark randomized controlled trials that demonstrated, among other important findings, that en bloc resection of axillary lymph nodes and radical surgery in all women with breast cancer were not associated with better outcomes.

A critical notion that emerged out of these trials and other discussions was that standardizing the classification of specific cancers into separate stages was important for both prognostic and treatment purposes, and nodal status was an integral component of overall stage. In 1959, 6 founding organizations (the American Cancer Society, American College of Surgeons [ACS], American Society of Clinical Oncology [ASCO], Centers for Disease Control and Prevention, National Cancer Institute [NCI], and College of American Pathologists) convened to launch the American Joint Committee on Cancer (AJCC).[5] The objective of the AJCC was to define cancer-staging groups that optimized prognostic estimates based on tumor size, nodal status, and presence of distant metastasis. Standardizing cancer staging has allowed researchers to reliably evaluate many important questions in cancer surgery, including those specific to the optimal extent of lymphadenectomy.

COLON CANCER

Colon cancer is the fourth most common malignancy diagnosed in the United States, and approximately 80% of patients present with potentially resectable disease. Nodal metastases have long been recognized as the most important factor that predicts long-term survival[1] and are an important determinant in the decision to administer adjuvant chemotherapy. With the demonstration of highly effective systemic therapies for colon cancer over the last decade, it is essential to ensure that all patients who would benefit from such treatment are well staged and have access to these therapies.[6]

Studies have shown an improvement in disease-specific and overall survival when increasing numbers of lymph nodes are examined for colon cancer.[7–9] This improvement in outcomes is due in part to stage migration or more accurate staging that allows for increased use of adjuvant chemotherapy. Although estimates have varied widely, numerous studies and consensus guidelines (eg, College of American Pathologists Consensus Statement 1999[10]) have suggested that the examination of 12 regional lymph nodes is a reasonable minimum for adequate nodal evaluation of colon cancer.[11–13] Despite these findings, population-based assessments have shown that most patients in the United States do not have 12 or more nodes examined.[14–16] This assessment, in part, motivated the ACS, ASCO, and National Comprehensive Cancer Network (NCCN) to harmonize a quality measure requiring the resection and pathologic examination of 12 or more lymph nodes for the evaluation of colon cancer.[16,17] Subsequently, the National Quality Forum endorsed the 12-node measure for quality surveillance.[12]

Using data from the National Cancer Data Base (NCDB) and examining treatment of colon cancer in patients who underwent colectomy at 1296 hospitals, Bilimoria and colleagues[15] found that although the proportion of compliant hospitals increased considerably during the study period, 60% of hospitals failed to comply with the 12-node measure (**Fig. 1**). Prior studies conducted at the level of individual patients have demonstrated that approximately 37% to 50% of patients with colon cancer in the United States have 12 or more nodes examined.[14] Nodal evaluation is likely to improve further with the development of the 12-node measure for quality, as physicians and hospitals recognize that the requirement to examine 12 or more nodes may affect referral and reimbursement. This quality measure will also soon be reported publicly.

RECTAL CANCER

Rectal cancer exemplifies the Halstedian theory of cancer progression, that is, spreading in an orderly manner via surrounding lymphatic channels. However, lymph node resection in rectal carcinoma presents some distinct challenges. In 1979, Heald[18] first described the total mesorectal excision (TME), a procedure that removes

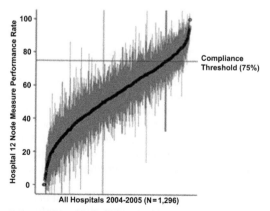

Fig. 1. Proportion of Commission on Cancer hospitals meeting the 12-node measure performance rates from 2004 to 2005. (*From* Bilimoria KY, Bentrem DJ, Stewart AK, et al. Lymph node evaluation as a colon cancer quality measure: a national hospital report card. J Natl Cancer Inst 2008;100(18):1314; with permission.)

all regional lymph nodes in the mesorectum, since demonstrated to substantially decrease tumor recurrence and improve survival.[19] However, the adequacy of TME may vary considerably even among experienced surgeons. For example, in the Dutch TME trial,[20] even after surgical standardization was performed among all participating surgeons, the quality of TME specimens was inadequate in as many as one-third of patients who were treated with abdominoperineal resection.[21]

Another challenge in rectal cancer is determining the optimal number of lymph nodes that should be examined after neoadjuvant therapy. Although treatment guidelines for rectal cancer are similar to those of colon cancer indicating that at least 12 nodes should be examined,[5,11] patients with T3/T4 or N+ rectal cancers should receive neoadjuvant therapy. Because preoperative chemoradiotherapy may reduce the number of nodes available for examination, the precise number of nodes, if any, that should be optimally removed is unclear.[22] Estimates in the literature are variable, ranging between 0 and 20, and there is yet to be a clear consensus.[23–25] For example, in a recent report from the MD Anderson Cancer Center, over a 14-year period Tsai and colleagues[25] found that when 7 or more nodes were examined, patients showed decreased tumor recurrence and improved cancer-specific survival. By contrast, Rullier and colleagues[24] failed to find any association between the number of nodes examined and survival. Although this issue remains controversial, it is clear that staging of lymph nodes is important whether or not neoadjuvant therapy is administered. At present, the authors continue to advocate that surgeons and pathologists continue to follow guidelines recommending the examination of at least 12 lymph nodes.

Similar to colon cancer, in rectal cancer, hospital-level performance with respect to lymph node examination rates is variable. In one of the few population-based studies evaluating the number of patients with colorectal cancer with at least 12 lymph nodes examined, Baxter and colleagues[14] found that rectal cancer was an independent factor associated with decreased lymph node harvests. The study also reported that overall only 23% of patients with stage I cancer received adequate lymph node evaluation. Nevertheless, rectal carcinoma poses unique challenges, and further research is required to elucidate these controversies.

PANCREATIC CANCER

Pancreatic cancer continues to pose substantial diagnostic and treatment challenges. Among GI cancers, pancreatic cancer has one of the worst prognosis and is most commonly diagnosed at later stages of the disease when curative resection is not possible. Nonetheless, in patients who have resectable disease, staging of lymph nodes has been shown to be one of the most important prognostic factors.[26] Similar to other GI malignancies, it is unclear if this survival advantage reflects stage migration or whether there is a therapeutic benefit of lymphadenectomy. Establishing lymph node involvement is especially important for stratifying pancreatic cancer in clinical trials. Moreover, Tomlinson and colleagues[27] demonstrated that well-staged node-negative patients had a median survival benefit of 8 months more than less-well-staged node-negative patients (**Fig. 2**). This improvement of survival is greater than with any adjuvant therapy.

Several studies have also investigated the optimal extent of lymphadenectomy that should be performed in pancreatic cancer. One study, performed by Schwarz and colleagues[28] using Surveillance, Epidemiology, and End Results (SEER) data from 1973 to 2000, demonstrated that resecting 10 to 15 nodes in node-negative patients improved survival. Two separate SEER studies[27,29] using different methodologies and

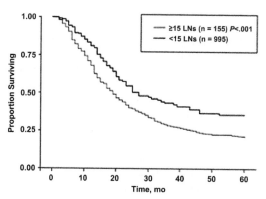

Fig. 2. Kaplan-Meier survival curves in patients with node-negative pancreatic cancer with 15 or more lymph nodes and less than 15 lymph nodes, examined after pancreatectomy. (*From* Tomlinson JS, Jain S, Bentrem DJ, et al. Accuracy of staging node-negative pancreas cancer: a potential quality measure. Arch Surg 2007;142(8):770 [discussion: 773–4]; with permission.)

patient populations essentially confirmed this threshold of 10 to 15 nodes. At present, both the NCCN and the AJCC support this recommendation.

Despite the importance of staging lymph nodes, evidence suggests that most hospitals in the United States do not meet the benchmark of 15 lymph nodes. In a 2008 study from the NCDB, Bilimoria and colleagues[30] showed that in 2004, only 16.4% of patients with pancreatic cancer had at least 15 nodes examined after surgery (**Fig. 3**). In this study, the median number of nodes examined was only 7, far fewer than what is recommended. Patients were found to be significantly more likely to have an adequate resection at NCCN-NCI centers, yet even at these experienced centers, rates of lymph node examination remained low at only 27%. Consistent with this study, a separate report using SEER data from 1988 to 2003 found that approximately 70% of patients had fewer than 15 lymph nodes examined after surgical resection.[29] These statistics are striking in a disease for which the only hope for cure is surgery. Although high-volume centers met the benchmark of 15 lymph nodes more frequently, there is still substantial room for improvement.

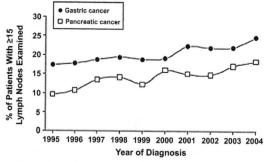

Fig. 3. Trends in lymph node evaluation for gastric and pancreatic cancers from the NCDB (1995–2004). (*From* Bilimoria KY, Talamonti MS, Wayne JD, et al. Effect of hospital type and volume on lymph node evaluation for gastric and pancreatic cancer. Arch Surg 2008;143(7):672 [discussion: 678]; with permission.)

GASTRIC CANCER

The presence of positive lymph nodes in gastric cancer has long been recognized as one of the most important prognostic factors. In 1889, Mikulicz, a Polish-Austrian surgeon in step with the Halstedian theory of cancer progression, was one of the first investigators to promote the importance of extended lymphadenectomy in gastric cancer.[31] Like Halsted, Mikulicz believed that cancer required aggressive locoregional surgery if there was to be any hope for cure.

Yet, more than a century later, the extent of lymphadenectomy in gastric cancer remains one of the most controversial debates in GI oncology. Principally there are 3 main lymph node resection categories: D0 (incomplete removal of perigastric nodes), D1 (complete removal of perigastric nodes), and D2 (extended lymphadenectomy, including common hepatic, left gastric, celiac, and splenic lymph nodes with or without splenectomy). The debate essentially echoes the Halstedian versus Fisherian arguments. Proponents of the D2 resection believe that cancer cells spread in an orderly manner, passing through lymphatic vessels; thus removal of all this tissue should portend a survival advantage. Opponents believe that this extensive surgical procedure only adds potential morbidity, not any survival advantage, and is necessary only for staging purposes. Many trials have attempted to address this issue but with variable results.[32–36] Recently, the long-term results of the Dutch randomized trial that supported the D2 resection were reported,[36] which are consistent with current consensus guidelines.[11]

A related issue is the determination of the optimal number of lymph nodes to be resected and evaluated during gastrectomy. Several analyses have addressed this issue, and it seems that evaluating at least 15 lymph nodes provides a reliable estimate of the pathologic N stage and is consistent with current guideline algorithms.[11,36–39] According to a study by Karpeh and colleagues,[37] it was not the location of positive lymph nodes that was important but simply the overall number of positive nodes.

Few studies have evaluated performance with respect to the benchmark of 15 lymph nodes. Bilimoria and colleagues,[30] in a study from the NCDB that included more than 3000 patients, found that the median number of nodes examined was only 7, but the number was higher in NCCN-NCI hospitals than in community hospitals (12 vs 6). In addition, this study reported that only 23.2% of patients undergoing gastrectomy had at least 15 nodes examined (see **Fig. 2**). In a separate population-based study using SEER data, the median number of nodes was 10, and only 32% of patients underwent an adequate lymph node evaluation.[40] However, other reports from high-volume specialty centers have documented evaluation of more than 15 lymph nodes in nearly 80% of patients.[37] Given these data, most patients are not being adequately staged, which may partially explain some of the survival differences between specialized cancer centers and community centers.

ESOPHAGEAL CANCER

In esophageal cancer, the extent of lymphadenectomy has important prognostic and therapeutic implications; however, a clear lymph node threshold has not been defined. The studies performed have been heterogeneous, with variable study inclusion and exclusion criteria. In addition, as with other GI malignancies, lymph node metastases may simply be a marker of systemic disease. Nevertheless, positive lymph nodes are powerful prognostic indicators, and numerous reports now show the benefits of adequate lymph node examination, with thresholds ranging from 10 to 40 nodes.[41–45] The NCCN[11] currently recommends that at least 15 nodes be examined, and the AJCC

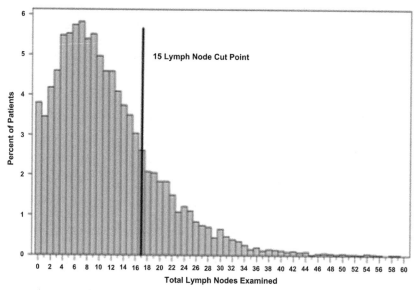

Fig. 4. Proportion of patients receiving lymph node evaluation of at least 15 nodes from 1998 to 2007.

staging manual identifies 4 distinct groups (N0–N3) of nodal metastasis, highlighting the need for adequate nodal examination for staging accuracy.[46]

Similar to rectal cancer, most patients with stage II and III esophageal cancers are treated with neoadjuvant therapy,[47] yet almost all studies examining lymph node thresholds exclude these patients from analysis.[43] In a recent study, Solomon and colleagues[48] examined the interaction of preoperative therapy and lymph node evaluation, and found that patients had the best survival if they received both adequate lymph node resection (defined as ≥18 nodes in this study) and neoadjuvant therapy. Nevertheless, no study has adequately examined the optimal number of nodes that should be removed after neoadjuvant therapy or the quality of lymph node examination in the United States. However, recent work from the NCDB Participant Use File suggests that fewer than one-third of patients and less than 1 in 10 hospitals met the benchmark of examining 15 or more nodes (**Fig. 4**), clearly demonstrating a gap in the quality of cancer care at many Commission on Cancer centers in the United States.[49]

SUMMARY

About 25% of all cancer-related deaths are a result of a GI malignancy, and the presence of lymph node metastases is one of the most powerful indicators of poor survival. Only by accurate staging through adequate lymph node evaluation can patients be correctly identified to receive appropriate postoperative adjuvant therapies and optimally stratified for clinical trials. In addition, although there is still debate between the Halstedian and Fisherian philosophies regarding the extent of lymphadenectomy, it remains an important part of cancer staging. Given the current evidence, there appears to be a concerning lack of adequate lymph node examination in the United States. Providers will soon be publicly evaluated and compensated based on quality metrics, such as the quality of lymph node staging, and therefore this problem must be addressed. To provide this type of information, organizations such as the ACS Cancer

Programs are beginning to develop rapid feedback mechanisms to cancer centers so that hospitals can identify and address potential problems early.[50] Moreover, future studies should investigate both structural and process-related factors that could potentially improve the quality of lymphadenectomy at poorly performing centers.

REFERENCES

1. Jemal A, Siegel R, Xu J, et al. Cancer statistics, 2010. CA Cancer J Clin 2010; 60(5):277–300.
2. Senthil M, Trisal V, Paz IB, et al. Prediction of the adequacy of lymph node retrieval in colon cancer by hospital type. Arch Surg 2010;145(9):840–3.
3. Halsted WS. I. The results of radical operations for the cure of carcinoma of the breast. Ann Surg 1907;46(1):1–19.
4. Fisher B, Fisher ER. Transmigration of lymph nodes by tumor cells. Science 1966; 152(727):1397–8.
5. American Joint Committee on Cancer (AJCC). Available at: http://www.cancerstaging. org/staging/index.html. Accessed August 1, 2011.
6. Benson AB 3rd. New approaches to the adjuvant therapy of colon cancer. Oncologist 2006;11(9):973–80.
7. Swanson RS, Compton CC, Stewart AK, et al. The prognosis of T3N0 colon cancer is dependent on the number of lymph nodes examined. Ann Surg Oncol 2003;10(1):65–71.
8. Wong JH, Severino R, Honnebier MB, et al. Number of nodes examined and staging accuracy in colorectal carcinoma. J Clin Oncol 1999;17(9):2896–900.
9. Chang GJ, Rodriguez-Bigas MA, Skibber JM, et al. Lymph node evaluation and survival after curative resection of colon cancer: systematic review. J Natl Cancer Inst 2007;99(6):433–41.
10. Compton CC, Fielding LP, Burgart LJ, et al. Prognostic factors in colorectal cancer. College of American Pathologists Consensus Statement 1999. Arch Pathol Lab Med 2000;124(7):979–94.
11. The National Comprehensive Cancer Network Guidelines in Oncology. Available at: http://www.nccn.org. Accessed August 1, 2011.
12. National Quality Forum. At least 12 regional lymph nodes are removed and pathologically examined for resected colon cancer. Available at: http://www.qualityforum. org/MeasureDetails.aspx?actid=0&SubmissionId=455#k=colon. Accessed May 5, 2011.
13. American College of Surgeons, Cancer Programs: Cancer Program Practice Profile Reports (CP3R). Available at: http://www.facs.org/cancer/ncdb/cp3r.html. Accessed August 8, 2011.
14. Baxter NN, Virnig DJ, Rothenberger DA, et al. Lymph node evaluation in colorectal cancer patients: a population-based study. J Natl Cancer Inst 2005; 97(3):219–25.
15. Bilimoria KY, Bentrem DJ, Stewart AK, et al. Lymph node evaluation as a colon cancer quality measure: a national hospital report card. J Natl Cancer Inst 2008; 100(18):1310–7.
16. Rajput A, Romanus D, Weiser MR, et al. Meeting the 12 lymph node (LN) benchmark in colon cancer. J Surg Oncol 2010;102(1):3–9.
17. American College of Surgeons, Cancer Programs. CoC Quality of Care Measures: National Quality Forum Endorsed Commission on Cancer Measures for Quality of Cancer Care for Breast and Colorectal Cancers. Available at: http://www.facs. org/cancer/qualitymeasures.html. Accessed May 2, 2011.

18. Heald RJ. A new approach to rectal cancer. Br J Hosp Med 1979;22(3):277–81.
19. Kapiteijn E, Putter H, van de Velde CJ. Impact of the introduction and training of total mesorectal excision on recurrence and survival in rectal cancer in The Netherlands. Br J Surg 2002;89(9):1142–9.
20. Kapiteijn E, Marijnen CA, Nagtegaal ID, et al. Preoperative radiotherapy combined with total mesorectal excision for resectable rectal cancer. N Engl J Med 2001;345(9):638–46.
21. Nagtegaal ID, van de Velde CJ, Marijnen CA, et al. Low rectal cancer: a call for a change of approach in abdominoperineal resection. J Clin Oncol 2005;23(36): 9257–64.
22. Baxter NN, Morris AM, Rothenberger DA, et al. Impact of preoperative radiation for rectal cancer on subsequent lymph node evaluation: a population-based analysis. Int J Radiat Oncol Biol Phys 2005;61(2):426–31.
23. Luna-Perez P, Rodriguez-Ramirez S, Alvarado I, et al. Prognostic significance of retrieved lymph nodes per specimen in resected rectal adenocarcinoma after preoperative chemoradiation therapy. Arch Med Res 2003; 34(4):281–6.
24. Rullier A, Laurent C, Capdepont M, et al. Lymph nodes after preoperative chemoradiotherapy for rectal carcinoma: number, status, and impact on survival. Am J Surg Pathol 2008;32(1):45–50.
25. Tsai CJ, Crane CH, Skibber JM, et al. Number of lymph nodes examined and prognosis among pathologically lymph node-negative patients after preoperative chemoradiation therapy for rectal adenocarcinoma. Cancer 2011;117(16):3713–22.
26. Brennan MF, Kattan MW, Klimstra D, et al. Prognostic nomogram for patients undergoing resection for adenocarcinoma of the pancreas. Ann Surg 2004; 240(2):293–8.
27. Tomlinson JS, Jain S, Bentrem DJ, et al. Accuracy of staging node-negative pancreas cancer: a potential quality measure. Arch Surg 2007;142(8):767–73 [discussion: 773–4].
28. Schwarz RE, Smith DD. Extent of lymph node retrieval and pancreatic cancer survival: information from a large US population database. Ann Surg Oncol 2006;13(9):1189–200.
29. Slidell MB, Chang DC, Cameron JL, et al. Impact of total lymph node count and lymph node ratio on staging and survival after pancreatectomy for pancreatic adenocarcinoma: a large, population-based analysis. Ann Surg Oncol 2008; 15(1):165–74.
30. Bilimoria KY, Talamonti MS, Wayne JD, et al. Effect of hospital type and volume on lymph node evaluation for gastric and pancreatic cancer. Arch Surg 2008;143(7): 671–8 [discussion: 678].
31. Olch PD. Johann von Mikulicz-Radecki. Ann Surg 1960;152:923–6.
32. Bonenkamp JJ, Hermans J, Sasako M, et al. Extended lymph-node dissection for gastric cancer. N Engl J Med 1999;340(12):908–14.
33. Bonenkamp JJ, Songun I, Hermans J, et al. Randomised comparison of morbidity after D1 and D2 dissection for gastric cancer in 996 Dutch patients. Lancet 1995; 345(8952):745–8.
34. McCulloch P, Nita ME, Kazi H, et al. Extended versus limited lymph nodes dissection technique for adenocarcinoma of the stomach. Cochrane Database Syst Rev 2004;(4):CD001964.
35. Cuschieri A, Weeden S, Fielding J, et al. Patient survival after D1 and D2 resections for gastric cancer: long-term results of the MRC randomized surgical trial. Surgical Co-operative Group. Br J Cancer 1999;79(9–10):1522–30.

36. Songun I, Putter H, Kranenbarg EM, et al. Surgical treatment of gastric cancer: 15-year follow-up results of the randomised nationwide Dutch D1D2 trial. Lancet Oncol 2010;11(5):439–49.

37. Karpeh MS, Leon L, Klimstra D, et al. Lymph node staging in gastric cancer: is location more important than number? An analysis of 1,038 patients. Ann Surg 2000;232(3):362–71.

38. Lee HK, Yang HK, Kim WH, et al. Influence of the number of lymph nodes examined on staging of gastric cancer. Br J Surg 2001;88(10):1408–12.

39. Bouvier AM, Haas O, Piard F, et al. How many nodes must be examined to accurately stage gastric carcinomas? Results from a population based study. Cancer 2002;94(11):2862–6.

40. Baxter NN, Tuttle TM. Inadequacy of lymph node staging in gastric cancer patients: a population-based study. Ann Surg Oncol 2005;12(12):981–7.

41. Hofstetter W, Correa AM, Bekele N, et al. Proposed modification of nodal status in AJCC esophageal cancer staging system. Ann Thorac Surg 2007;84(2):365–73 [discussion: 374–5].

42. Mariette C, Piessen G, Briez N, et al. The number of metastatic lymph nodes and the ratio between metastatic and examined lymph nodes are independent prognostic factors in esophageal cancer regardless of neoadjuvant chemoradiation or lymphadenectomy extent. Ann Surg 2008;247(2):365–71.

43. Rizk NP, Ishwaran H, Rice TW, et al. Optimum lymphadenectomy for esophageal cancer. Ann Surg 2010;251(1):46–50.

44. Peyre CG, Hagen JA, DeMeester SR, et al. The number of lymph nodes removed predicts survival in esophageal cancer: an international study on the impact of extent of surgical resection. Ann Surg 2008;248(4):549–56.

45. Barbour AP, Rizk NP, Gonen M, et al. Lymphadenectomy for adenocarcinoma of the gastroesophageal junction (GEJ): impact of adequate staging on outcome. Ann Surg Oncol 2007;14(2):306–16.

46. AJCC cancer staging manual. 7th edition. Chicago: Springer; 2010.

47. Merkow RP, Bilimoria KY, McCarter MD, et al. Use of multimodality neoadjuvant therapy for esophageal cancer in the United States: assessment of 987 hospitals. Ann Surg Oncol 2012;19(2):357–64.

48. Solomon N, Zhuge Y, Cheung M, et al. The roles of neoadjuvant radiotherapy and lymphadenectomy in the treatment of esophageal adenocarcinoma. Ann Surg Oncol 2010;17(3):791–803.

49. Merkow RP, Bilimoria KY, Bentrem DJ, et al. Variation in lymph node examination after esophagectomy for cancer in the United States. Arch Surg, in press.

50. Raval MV, Bilimoria KY, Stewart AK, et al. Using the NCDB for cancer care improvement: an introduction to available quality assessment tools. J Surg Oncol 2009;99(8):488–90.

Racial Differences and Disparities in Cancer Care and Outcomes

Where's the Rub?

Nestor F. Esnaola, MD, MPH, MBA[a],*, Marvella E. Ford, PhD[b]

KEYWORDS

- White - Black - Race - Differences - Disparities - Cancer

KEY POINTS

- Racial differences in outcomes have been reported for almost all cancer types.
- The preponderance of the medical literature to date suggests that black-white differences in cancer outcomes are largely explained by failure to provide suitable cancer care rather than by racial differences in stage at presentation, tumor biology, or response to treatments.
- Studies using novel research methodologies and accounting for sociodemographic, physician, and hospital factors are needed to identify potentially modifiable patient, physician, and health care system factors that may underlie persistent racial disparities in receipt and quality of surgical and adjuvant therapy.
- Ongoing efforts to improve access to care, enhance diversity in the surgical workforce, navigate minority cancer patients through the health care system, and enhance adherence to cancer-specific best practices are warranted.

RACIAL DIFFERENCES IN CANCER OUTCOMES: SCOPE OF THE PROBLEM

Although racial differences in outcomes have been reported for almost all cancer types, this article focuses primarily on the 3 leading causes of cancer death in the United States for which the standard of care is well defined and surgical resection is the cornerstone of therapy: invasive breast cancer, non–small cell lung cancer

This work was supported by a grant from the Resource Center for Minority Aging Research (MUSC) and an American Cancer Society Institutional Research Grant from the Hollings Cancer Center (MUSC).
The authors have nothing to disclose.
[a] Division of Surgical Oncology, Department of Surgery, Medical University of South Carolina, 25 Courtenay Drive, Suite 7018, Charleston, SC 29425, USA; [b] Division of Biostatistics and Epidemiology, Department of Medicine, Medical University of South Carolina, 86 Jonathan Lucas Street, Charleston, SC 29425, USA
* Corresponding author.
E-mail address: esnaolan@musc.edu

Surg Oncol Clin N Am 21 (2012) 417–437
doi:10.1016/j.soc.2012.03.012
1055-3207/12/$ – see front matter © 2012 Published by Elsevier Inc.

(NSCLC), and colorectal cancer (**Table 1**).[1] Recent statistics indicate that age-adjusted breast cancer mortality rates are higher among black women than white women (**Table 2**).[1] Population-based studies suggest that although survival rates for women with breast cancer have improved over the past 2 decades, survival rates in black women have lagged behind, and the observed disparity is increasing.[2–4] Black men have a significantly higher incidence rate and are almost 1.5 times as likely to die from lung cancer and bronchus cancer than are white men.[1] Similarly, black men and black women have significantly higher cancer incidence rates and are approximately 1.5 more likely to die of colorectal cancer compared with their white counterparts.[1]

MECHANISMS UNDERLYING RACIAL DIFFERENCES IN CANCER OUTCOMES

Racial differences in cancer outcomes may be attributed to racial differences in stage at presentation, tumor biology, treatment efficacy, and/or failure to provide optimal cancer treatment.

Cancer Stage

Data from the National Cancer Institute (NCI) Surveillance, Epidemiology and End Results (SEER) program have persistently shown than blacks with breast cancer, lung cancer, and colorectal cancer are more likely to present with advanced disease compared with whites (**Fig. 1**).[1] Failure to uncover black-white differences in biologic and tumor characteristics suggests that discrepancies in routine cancer screening between races may be involved.[5–14] Studies further suggest that the effect of race on stage at presentation may be confounded by socioeconomic factors, including education, income, and insurance status.[10,15] Irrespective of the mechanisms involved, black-white differences in cancer survival persist even when controlling for stage at presentation, suggesting that other factors likely account for observed racial differences in cancer outcomes (**Fig. 2**).[1]

Tumor Biology

Although racial differences in tumor biology (and natural history) may contribute to differences in cancer outcomes, their influence and true impact on outcomes remains controversial. In a study combining breast cancer incidence data from various SEER registries and mortality data from the National Center for Health Statistics, breast cancer mortality rates were similar for blacks and whites until the late 1970s, after which time the mortality rates among black women increased.[16] This observation was associated with

Table 1
Estimated new cancer cases and deaths (by gender), United States, 2011

	Men			Women		
	No. of Cases	% of Cases	Rank	No. of Cases	% of Cases	Rank
Estimated New Cases						
Breast	—	—	—	230,480	30	1
Lung and bronchus	115,060	14	2	106,070	14	2
Colon and rectum	71,850	9	3	69,360	9	3
Estimated Deaths						
Breast	—	—	—	71,340	26	2
Lung and bronchus	85,600	11	1	39,520	15	1
Colon and rectum	25,250	8	3	24,130	9	3

Table 2
Incidence and mortality rates (by gender and race), United States, 2011

	Men		Women	
	White	Black	White	Black
Incidence rates				
Breast	—	—	121.9	114.6
Lung and bronchus	84.3	103.5	57.0	51.8
Colon and rectum	56.1	67.2	41.4	50.7
Mortality rates				
Breast	—	—	23.4	32.4
Lung and bronchus	68.3	87.5	41.6	39.6
Colon and rectum	20.6	30.5	14.4	21.0

an increase in the calendar period mortality curves for blacks but not the birth cohort curves (which reflect differences in risk factors), suggesting that the greater mortality rate in blacks may have been attributable to differences in access to care or response to new treatments during this period. Studies also suggest that there are no apparent racial differences in the biologic aggressiveness, tumor characteristics, or efficacy of treatments for colorectal cancer.[9,13,17,18] In the NCI Black/White Cancer Survival Study, the distribution of colon cancers by anatomic location, histology, and grade did not differ by race.[13]

Treatment Toxicity and Efficacy

Treatment-related mortality
Several investigators have suggested that race is an independent predictor of poor outcomes after surgery.[19–23] In a study using Medicare data, black race was

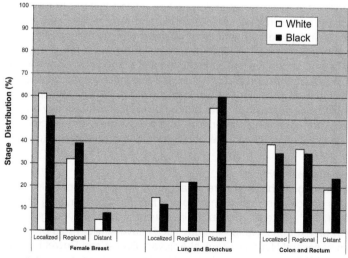

Fig. 1. Stage of diagnosis by cancer type and race; United States, 1999 to 2006. (*Data from* Siegel R, Ward E, Brawley O, et al. Cancer statistics, 2011: the impact of eliminating socioeconomic and racial disparities on premature cancer deaths. CA Cancer J Clin 2011;61(4): 212–36.)

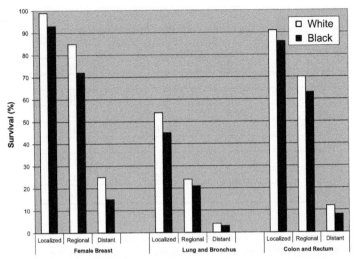

Fig. 2. Five-year relative survival rates by cancer type, stage, and race; United States, 1999 to 2006. (*Data from* Siegel R, Ward E, Brawley O, et al. Cancer statistics, 2011: the impact of eliminating socioeconomic and racial disparities on premature cancer deaths. CA Cancer J Clin 2011;61(4):212–36.)

associated with an increased risk of death after 7 of 8 major cardiovascular or cancer procedures (even when adjusting for comorbidity using administrative data codes).[22] This effect, however, was attenuated or nonexistent when controlling for the proportion of black patients treated at the operating hospitals.

In a more recent study using data from the National Surgery Quality Improvement Program (NSQIP) Patient Safety in Surgery Study, blacks were more likely to present with greater comorbidity and more likely to undergo emergency surgery than whites.[24] After controlling for all other patient/procedure-related factors, however, black race was associated with a higher risk of cardiac and renal postoperative occurrences but was not an independent predictor of overall morbidity or mortality.

With the exception of the NSQIP report, these studies have relied largely on administrative data sets, which are limited in the amount of clinical information available for accurate risk adjustment and can only be used to generate approximate measures of comorbidity, such as the Charlson Comorbidity Index (CCI).[25] The apparent adverse effects of black race on postoperative outcomes in these studies may be due to failure to fully control for underlying comorbidity and/or structures and processes of care at the hospitals at which patients were treated rather than race per se (discussed later).

Efficacy of adjuvant therapy

Many studies suggest that there are no apparent racial differences in the efficacy or effectiveness of local and/or systemic therapy for breast cancer, lung cancer, or colorectal cancer.[26–29] White women and black women with early-stage breast cancer treated with breast conservation therapy (BCT) have similar rates of local control.[30] An analysis of several National Surgical Adjuvant Breast and Bowel Project (NSABP) trials between 1982 and 1994 revealed no differences in disease-free survival between racial groups.[31] Survival in whites and blacks with early-stage NSCLC is similar after resection.[32,33] In patients with more advanced disease, race-related survival is also comparable after radiation and systemic therapy.[34,35] Reanalyses of randomized,

NSABP colorectal cancer adjuvant therapy trials revealed similar rates of nodal involvement and no black-white differences in disease-free survival.[17,18]

Failure to Provide Optimal Cancer Treatment

There is a growing body of literature suggesting that black-white differences in cancer outcomes may be explained by failure to provide suitable cancer care in blacks, due to either underuse of therapy and/or receipt of suboptimal therapy.[36]

Underuse of surgical resection

Surgical resection is the cornerstone of therapy in patients with nonmetastatic breast cancer, NSCLC, and colorectal cancer. Failure to perform resection in these patients represents a serious breach in the standard of care and poses a serious threat to patients' quality of life and long-term survival.

Although the majority of studies to date in breast cancer patients have focused primarily on black-white differences in the use of BCT, a 2002 report that linked data from the Metropolitan Detroit SEER registry to Michigan Medicaid enrollment files reported underuse of surgical resection among blacks with breast cancer.[29,37–41] In a multivariate analysis controlling for age, marital status, Medicaid enrollment, poverty status, and stage, black race was associated with an adjusted odds ratio (OR) of resection of 0.62 (95% CI, 0.42–0.90).[41] In a recent study using a large, population-based sample of women with nonmetastatic breast cancer, black race was associated with underuse of curative resection (94.9% vs 96.4%, $P<.001$).[42] Although black race had no apparent adverse effect on resection among rural patients, the adjusted OR for resection for urban black patients was 0.58 (95% CI, 0.41–0.82). These studies suggest that underuse of resection among urban black women with breast cancer is real and seems to extend across geographically diverse communities, independent of comorbidity or socioeconomic status (SES). Although the black-white differences in surgical resection rates in these studies are admittedly small, long-term, breast cancer survival is impossible without surgical resection. Therefore, even minor differences in surgical treatment can be considered clinically significant, particularly when surgery carries minimal risks to the patient.

Approximately one-third of patients with the most common type of lung cancer, NSCLC, present with early (stage I or II), potentially curable disease. If treated with resection, the 5-year survival rate of these patients approaches 40%. In contrast, the median survival of patients who are not resected or patients with locally advanced/metastatic disease is less than 1 year.[43] Several studies have reported lower rates of lung resection among blacks with NSCLC, even when controlling for stage at presentation. Greenwald and colleagues[44] reported that patients with stage I NSCLC in Detroit, San Francisco, and Seattle were less likely (by 12.7%) to undergo resection if they were black or of lower SES. In a seminal study using SEER-Medicare data from 1985 to 1993, the rate of surgery in black patients with stage I-II NSCLC was only 64.0% compared with 76.7% among whites ($P<.001$).[33] Black race was associated with a relative risk of resection of 0.54, even when controlling for the effects of age, gender, comorbidity, median income, and tumor stage. Overall, 5-year survival rates were lower for blacks compared with whites (26.4% vs 34.1%, $P<.001$). In contrast, the 5-year survival rates of black patients and white patients who underwent surgery were approximately similar (39.1 vs 42.9%, $P = .10$) as were survival rates among patients who did not undergo surgery (4% vs 5%, $P = .25$). The investigators concluded that the racial disparity in resection rates largely accounted for the lower survival rate among blacks in their study. In a more recent study of all cases of non-metastatic NSCLC reported to the South Carolina Central Cancer Registry between

1996 and 2002, overall use of surgical resection (across races) was lower than previously reported, and blacks were significantly less likely to undergo surgery compared with whites (44.7% vs 63.4%, P<.001).[45] After controlling for sociodemographics, comorbidity, and tumor factors, the adjusted OR for resection for blacks was 0.43 (95% CI, 0.34–0.55).

Several recent studies using state cancer registry data, SEER data, and the National Cancer Data Base (NCDB) have also reported lower rates of definitive resection among blacks with resectable colon and rectal cancers.[5,14] A study of more than 80,000 Medicare beneficiaries with colorectal cancer reported that only 68% of blacks underwent surgical resection compared with 78% of whites.[46] A study using SEER data reported rates of surgery of 94% among black patients with stage II-III rectal cancer compared with 96% among white patients.[5,8] In a more recent study, underuse of surgery was greater among blacks with rectal cancer (82.0% vs 89.3% in whites, P<.001) compared with blacks with colon cancer (92.9% vs 94.5% in whites, P<.001).[47] In a nationwide, hospital-based sample of 35,695 patients with rectal cancer treated between 2003 and 2005 culled from the NCDB, only 85.1% percent of blacks underwent definitive resection compared with 90.7% of whites.[14] Black race was independently associated with underuse of surgery on multivariate analysis (OR 0.62; 95% CI, 0.54–0.71) even when controlling for comorbidity and SES/insurance status.

Underuse of adjuvant therapy

In addition to underuse of surgical resection, underuse of adjuvant radiation and/or systemic therapy in blacks with nonmetastatic breast cancer, NSCLC, and colorectal cancer may partly explain observed differences in survival. Despite similar rates of comorbidity, insurance coverage, and oncologic consultation, women with early-stage breast cancer from minority groups were half as likely to receive adjuvant therapy than were whites.[48] Several population-based studies using SEER data have also reported lower rates of adjuvant radiation therapy after BCT.[49,50]

A study that used SEER data reported that black race was associated with underuse of adjuvant radiotherapy, contradicting a previous analysis that used SEER-Medicare data.[5,51] In a more recent study from the NCDB, however, there was no association between race and receipt or type of adjuvant therapy.[14] A study of 3 population-based databases in California similarly found no association between race/ethnicity and use of adjuvant therapy when controlling for comorbidity, education, and poverty status.[52] Taken as a whole, these studies suggest that whatever race-related barriers to surgical care may exist among black patients with rectal cancer, they do not seem to affect the quality of their nonsurgical cancer care.

Factors underlying underuse of cancer treatment
Patient factors

Misconceptions about cancer and its treatment Patients' misconceptions about cancer and its treatment may adversely impact their willingness to undergo surgery. In a national telephone survey, the misconception, "Treating cancer with surgery can cause it to spread throughout the body," was endorsed by 41% of respondents.[53] A significant proportion of respondents endorsed other misconceptions, including "The medical industry is withholding a cure for cancer from the public to increase profits" (27%); "All you need to beat cancer is a positive attitude, not treatment" (11%); and "Cancer is something that cannot be effectively treated" (13%). Respondents who were older, nonwhite, Southern, or indicated being less informed about cancer endorsed the most misconceptions.

In a related study of patients being treated at pulmonary and lung cancer clinics in Philadelphia, Los Angeles, and Charleston, 38% of patients stated that they believed that air exposure at surgery caused tumor spread and that black race was the most significant predictor of this belief; 19% of black patients stated that this belief was a reason for avoiding surgery, and 14% stated that they would not accept their physicians' reassurance that the belief was false.[54] In a recent prospective cohort study of patients with early-stage lung cancer from North Carolina and South Carolina, 45% of patients agreed with this belief and endorsement of this belief was significantly associated with subsequent failure to undergo surgery.[55]

Patient preferences Patients' beliefs and preferences may affect their decision to undergo cancer treatment. Patients facing a tradeoff between quantity and quality of life may (paradoxically) opt to forgo potentially curative surgery. In one study, 20% of subjects facing T3 laryngeal cancer opted for radiation therapy (and a lower probability of survival, 30%–40%) over laryngectomy (and a higher probability of survival, 60%) to preserve their speech.[56]

In a prospective study of black veterans and white veterans with carotid stenosis faced with the prospect of carotid angiography and carotid endarterectomy, blacks expressed higher aversion to surgery than whites.[57] During follow-up, 20% of whites and 14% of blacks underwent endarterectomy, and highest aversion quartile was associated with a lower likelihood of undergoing surgery, even when accounting for clinical appropriateness. In a secondary analysis, increased age, black race, no previous surgery, lower level of chance locus of control, less trust of physicians, and less social support were associated with greater likelihood of surgery risk aversion.[58]

In a 2004 study, blacks with colorectal cancer were more likely to refuse surgery when reasons for nonreceipt of surgery were analyzed using the SEER database.[59] Concerns or fears about receiving a permanent stoma may affect patients' willingness to pursue surgical consultation and/or follow-up with recommended surgery (which may explain why blacks with nonmetastatic rectal cancer were more likely to forgo radical resection and opt for local excision in a recent study from the NCDB).[14] In a prospective cohort study of patients with early-stage lung cancer, the feeling that quality of life would be worse 1 year after lung cancer surgery was significantly higher among blacks than whites (42% vs 34%) and was associated with subsequent failure to undergo surgical resection.[55]

Health care system factors

Access to care Black-white differences in cancer care and outcomes may be partly explained by differences in access to care. In the Community Tracking Study Physician Survey, black Medicare beneficiaries were more likely to be cared for by physicians who were less well trained clinically and had more limited access to important clinical resources (eg, specialists, high-quality imaging, high-quality ancillary services, and nonemergency hospital admissions) than physicians who treated white patients.[60] Lack of a regular source of health care was recently shown to be associated with underuse of surgical resection in patients with early-stage lung cancer, particularly among blacks.[55]

Although underuse of surgery could also be related to lower referral rates for surgical consultation among blacks, the widely varying black-white differences in resection rates in patients with breast cancer, lung cancer, and colorectal cancer argue against systematic under-referral of blacks. In addition, a recent study showed that black race was a powerful, negative predictor of surgical resection even when the analysis was limited to patients who had received surgical consultation and been previously staged with mediastinoscopy.[33]

To what extent does equal access to appropriate cancer care reduce black-white differences in treatment and outcomes? Dominitz and colleagues analyzed the effect of black race on surgery and adjuvant therapy in a cohort of 3176 colorectal cancer patients treated within the Veterans Administration (VA) equal access health care system.[61] Irrespective of SES, blacks and whites had similar rates of surgery, radiation therapy, and chemotherapy (likely because referral patterns and payments were not barriers to care) and survival was similar across races. Equal health care coverage (ie, insurance), however, may not be sufficient to ensure equal access to care. Rogers and colleagues[12] analyzed the effect of race on colorectal cancer outcomes in a population of elderly Tennesseans who were dually enrolled in both Medicaid and Medicare. Although there was no racial difference in overall mortality in a multivariate analysis controlling for comorbidity, stage, and treatment, only 86% of blacks received surgical therapy compared with 91% of whites ($P = .02$).

Physician-patient communication In a recent report from the cancer registry at the Henry Ford Health System in Detroit, black race had no apparent effect on the odds of being offered surgery for early-stage NSCLC (after controlling for comorbidity, pulmonary function, and tumor stage) but did have a negative effect on the rate at which surgery was declined by patients (OR 4.1; 95% CI, 0.34–0.55).[62] In another study, black patients evaluated by a surgeon were more likely to have a negative recommendation for surgery (71.4% vs 67.0%, $P<.05$) and more likely to refuse surgery compared with whites (3.4% vs 2.0%, $P = .013$), suggesting that that miscommunication or bias during the patient-physician encounter was likely involved.[33]

Several factors can influence patients' decisions to undergo treatment. In a study of patients with advanced lung cancer, their caregivers, and medical oncologists, all 3 groups ranked the oncologist's recommendation as the most important factor in decision making.[63] Patients and caregivers ranked faith in God second (above the ability of treatment to cure their cancer), whereas physicians ranked faith last. Patients who ranked faith first were less educated and may not have fully understood the technical aspects or risks/benefits of their cancer treatments. Failure by physicians to acknowledge their patients' strongly held beliefs might lead to unsatisfactory physician-patient interactions and suboptimal decision making. In a recent study of patients with early-stage lung cancer, patients who agreed with the statements, "faith alone cures disease" and "prayer will cure cancer," were less likely to receive subsequent surgical resection.[55] In addition, negative perceptions of physician-patient communication were associated with underuse of surgery across races.

In a recent analysis of audiotaped office visits between orthopedic surgeons and white versus black elderly patients, there were no significant differences in the content of various informed decision-making elements by race.[64] When the encounters were evaluated for 4 relationship-building components of communication, however, coder ratings were significantly lower for responsiveness, respectfulness, and listening in visits with black patients. Not surprisingly, black patients were significantly less satisfied with the encounters and their surgeons, even after controlling for potential confounders.

Physician beliefs and biases Persistent erroneous beliefs (reinforced by published reports) about the adverse effect of black race on surgical mortality and/or treatment efficacy may deter physicians from referring black patients with potentially curable cancers for surgical resection and/or adjuvant therapy.[22,65] Race and SES can also affect physicians' perceptions of patients and subsequent treatment recommendations. In a study of physicians from 8 New York hospitals, black patients of low SES were perceived more negatively by physicians during a postangiogram encounter.[66]

More specifically, blacks were more likely to be rated as less intelligent and educated, less likely to have poor social support, and more likely to be at risk for noncompliance.

Perceived racism by patients can also undermine the physician-patient relationship and ultimately result in mistrust and refusal to proceed with recommended treatments. In a survey of Medicare beneficiaries with localized breast cancer, blacks reported perceiving more ageism and racism in the health care system compared with whites, and ageism was associated with higher rates of mastectomy (compared with BCT) and omission of radiation after BCT.[67] In a study of patients from North Carolina and South Carolina, 62% of patients with early-stage lung cancer (73% of blacks and 50% of whites) agreed or mildly disagreed that patients receive worse care due to their race, and endorsement of this belief was associated with failure to undergo surgical resection for lung cancer. Furthermore, increasing distrust in the health care system was associated with an almost 2-fold increase in failure to undergo surgery.[55]

Factors underlying receipt of suboptimal cancer treatment

Physician knowledge and expertise Black patients with nonmetastatic cancer may be more likely to be referred to less experienced surgeons with worse perioperative outcomes. In a study from South Carolina, approximately 50% and 60% of lobectomies and pneumonectomies, respectively, for lung cancer were performed by general surgeons, and the perioperative mortality after lobectomy was significantly higher among patients treated by general surgeons (5.3% vs 3.0%, $P<.05$).[68] In a study analyzing the effect of surgeon volume versus hospital volume on outcomes after rectal cancer resection, surgeon volume was not associated with either 30-day mortality of rate of sphincter preservation.[69] Surgeon volume was strongly associated with 2-year mortality, however, and was a stronger predictor of long-term survival than hospital volume.

It is possible that black patients are more likely to be referred to less experienced surgeons, who in turn, may be more likely to recommend more radical (and perhaps less palatable) surgery. Some studies have reported lower rates of BCT and sphincter preservation in blacks with breast cancer and rectal cancer, respectively.[5,37,70] More recent work, however, has reported underuse of surgery but similar rates of sphincter preservation and adjuvant therapy among resected patients (suggesting that whatever barriers to care existed preoperatively, they did not seem to affect patients' intraoperative or postoperative care).[14]

Hospital factors In a recent report from California, blacks were significantly more likely to undergo surgery at low-volume centers for 6 of 10 operations (including lung cancer resection and pancreatectomy), even when controlling for comorbidity, insurance status, rural residence, and proximity to low-volume, medium-volume, and high-volume hospitals.[71] In addition, Medicaid patients (and uninsured patients) were also more likely to receive care at low-volume hospitals compared with Medicare patients. A recent analysis from the Nationwide Inpatient Sample also revealed that blacks who underwent lung resection were less likely to undergo surgery at high-volume hospitals and more likely to die postoperatively.[72] These and other studies risk-adjusted outcomes using administrative data and may have underestimated the true extent of comorbidity among precisely those patients who would have been more likely to receive care at low-volume centers (ie, minority and underfunded patients). In contrast, a report from the VA-NSQIP detected no statistically significant association between procedure or specialty volume and 30-day mortality rate when outcomes were risk-adjusted using the more rigorous NSQIP methodology.[73] "Evidence-based" hospital referral of selected patients to high-volume centers may not be practical, could exacerbate current racial disparities in access to care, and may inadvertently erode the level of surgical care at "low-volume" hospitals in rural and underserved areas.[74–77] Recent work suggests that surgeon volume is a better predictor of rectal cancer outcomes than hospital volume and that the effect of hospital surgical volume may be negligible in patients who receive standard adjuvant therapy.[69,78]

Hospital racial composition has also been shown to be associated with long-term outcomes in patients with breast cancer or colon cancer and attenuate the effect of individual patients' race within hospitals.[79] In a report of California Cancer Registry data, hospitals with a high Medicaid use rate (which cared for a disproportionate share of minority patients) had significantly higher 30-day and 1-year mortality rates compared with other hospitals.[80] Taken together, these studies suggest that financial and/or resource constraints at the hospitals at which minorities are cared for may result in suboptimal care and disparities in treatment and outcomes. In a study of Medicare beneficiaries with cancer, black race was associated with worse 1-year and 3-year survival rates (largely due to later stage of disease at presentation and underuse of cancer-directed surgery); black race had no apparent adverse effect on outcomes, however, when the analysis was restricted to patients treated at NCI-designated cancer centers.[81]

Moderators of receipt and quality of cancer treatment

Socioeconomic status To some extent, race is a sociocultural construct and its apparent effect on health care access, use, and outcomes can be mediated and moderated by SES.[82–84] In the NCI Black/White Cancer Survival Study, 26% of blacks lived at or below 125% of the poverty level income compared with only 9% of whites.[13] Increasing income was associated with decreasing all-cause mortality, and controlling for poverty status eradicated the apparent, increased risk of cancer death among black patients with stage II-III colon cancer. In a recent study, black race was a powerful predictor of underuse of surgical resection in patients with rectal cancer, but its adverse was limited to patients living in poverty.[47] Similarly, underuse of radiation after BCT was higher among blacks living greater distances from a cancer center or in areas of high poverty, whereas this effect was not seen in whites.[67] Despite similar health care coverage, patients living in poverty may have worse access to financial and/or social resources needed to successfully negotiate the costs and inherent complexities of multidisciplinary cancer care.

Urban/rural status Several studies have reported an association between rural residence and underuse of BCT (and adjuvant radiation after BCT) among women with invasive breast cancer.[39,70,85,86] In a recent study, rural residence was associated with underuse of surgery across races, and black race had no apparent adverse effect on resection rates among rural patients.[42] Rural women are less likely to have had a recent mammogram or breast examination compared with urban women (even when they report similar access to patient care) and tend to have more negative attitudes about breast cancer (despite having a similar knowledge base about the disease).[87] Rural residents also experience limited access to health care (due to longer travel distances), fewer benefits (such as paid sick leave), fewer support services (such as childcare), and scant access to specialty physicians, including surgeons.[67,88–91]

RESEARCH RECOMMENDATIONS AND FUTURE DIRECTIONS
Improve Collection of Sociodemographic Data

Although race data are available in Medicare claims for patients over age 65, they are less likely to be reliably or accurately recorded in younger patients. Given persistent racial disparities in cancer treatment and outcomes (and a growing body of literature suggesting that hospital racial composition may partly explain differences in outcomes previously attributed to patient race), it is imperative that race and ethnicity, ideally assessed by self-report, be accurately captured in the medical record.[82,92] Standardization of race and ethnicity codes (along federal standards published by the Office of Management and Budget) to meet "meaningful use" criteria for electronic health records will assist greatly in these efforts.

As discussed previously, the effects of race on health care access, use, and outcomes can be mediated and moderated by SES. Collection of socioeconomic data at the provider level and/or at the aggregate level is crucial.[93] Although not always correlated with individual level data, census tract or zip code level socioeconomic data can often be used to estimate and control for SES.[94]

Use Optimal Risk Adjustment Methodology

Risk-adjustment systems that rely on administrative data (including the CCI and its various modifications) rely on categories of comorbidities drawn from the *International Classification of Diseases, Ninth Revision, Clinical Modification* (*ICD-9-CM*) codes contained within hospital discharge/billing records.[25,95,96] *ICD-9-CM* codes often lack detailed, standardized definitions for use by medical record coders and are open to clinical and coding interpretation.[97] Comorbidities are often underreported using *ICD-9-CM* codes; thus, the sensitivity and positive predictive value of administrative data to identify preoperative risk factors is poor.[98]

The CCI was originally designed to empirically predict mortality among medical patients 1 year after admission.[25] Clinically based risk-adjustment methods (such as the ones used by the VA and ACS-NSQIP), alternatively, were specifically developed to identify independent predictors of 30-day surgical morbidity and mortality.[99,100] In a recent study comparing the ability of the two methods to predict 30-day mortality, the risk scores derived from each method were essentially uncorrelated and the predictive value of the NSQIP method far exceeded that of the CCI.[101] The ability of the CCI to correctly predict which patients would live or die after surgery was only marginally better than xpected by random chance. Nonetheless, the CCI has been widely used to control for comorbidity in several publications analyzing the effect of race, surgeon volume, and hospital volume on perioperative outcomes.[102–104]

Consider Alternative Research Methodologies

Qualitative research

Although further work using large clinical and administrative data sets is needed to determine to what extent racial differences in cancer treatment are explained by differences in sociodemographic characteristics, access to care, and physician/hospital characteristics, qualitative research exploring the relative effects of other (potentially modifiable) patient care–related, physician care–related, and health care system–related factors on patients' willingness to undergo recommended cancer treatments are also warranted. In response to a study demonstrating significant underuse of surgical therapy among black patients with localized NSCLC in South Carolina, the authors' program conducted a series of focus groups using white subjects and black subjects at risk for lung cancer to explore their perceptions of cancer and its treatment, their attitudes about physicians and the health care system, and their potential willingness to undergo surgical resection if diagnosed with lung cancer (Nestor Esnaola, MD, personal communication, 2011).[45] Among black subjects, willingness to undergo resection was negatively associated with reported fear of cancer and its treatment, a widely held belief that exposing cancer to air during surgery causes the cancer to spread ("once they open you up, all it [cancer] does is spread to the rest of the body"), mistrust of surgeons ("doctors just want to cut you"), and mistrust of the health care system. Black subjects also expressed a strong desire to receive better medical information ("good information and direction"), information about the risks and benefits of lung cancer surgery and alternative treatments ("being walked through the treatment process"), access to testimonials from patients who had successfully undergone surgical resection for lung cancer, help with financial barriers to surgery (eg, transportation barriers), and emotional support during the decision-making process ("receiving comfort would be helpful"). Similar work is needed to determine to what extent similar attitudes may underlie persistent underuse of surgical and/or adjuvant treatments for other cancer types.

Community-based participatory research

Community-based participatory research (CBPR) is a collaborative research approach whereby representatives from the communities affected by the issue being studied partner with organizations and researchers throughout the research process to facilitate and ensure (1) colearning/reciprocal transfer of expertise between groups, (2) shared decision making in the design and conduct of the research project, and (3) mutual ownership of the process and end product.[105] Knowledge and experiences shared via CBPR can strengthen the link between researchers and communities, refine research priorities, facilitate the creation of more culturally appropriate research instruments, and enhance the quantity and quality of collected data.

The Agency for Healthcare Research and Quality commissioned a study of the existing evidence on the conduct, process, and results of CBPR.[105] In the majority of the studies analyzed, communities were actively involved in recruiting and retaining participants. Communities were involved in setting research priorities/generating hypotheses and in study design/implementation in only half the studies, however. In the majority of the completed intervention studies, active community involvement resulted in enhanced intervention quality and enhanced recruitment; there was no evidence of diminished research quality resulting from CBPR.

HEALTH CARE POLICY IMPLICATIONS
Improve Access to Care

To what extent might a policy of providing insurance coverage to black, impoverished cancer patients mitigate racial disparities in treatment and outcomes? In response to the National Breast and Cervical Cancer Early Detection Program of 1991, several states established Best Chance Networks (BCNs) to contract with providers and facilities to provide funding for screening and diagnostic follow-up services to low-income women with abnormal breast screening results (and later, treatment coverage under Medicaid). Despite that approximately 60% of the women enrolled in South Carolina's BCN were black and/or resided in rural communities, a recent study reported persistent underuse of surgery among women with nonmetastatic breast cancer in these groups (including Medicaid patients).[42] In a study of elderly Tennesseans with colorectal cancer dually enrolled in both Medicaid and Medicare, blacks were significantly less likely to receive surgical resection compared with whites, despite having apparently identical health care coverage.[12] These studies suggest that although social programs to optimize access to care may be helpful, they are probably not sufficient (possibly due to persistent differences in access to care and specialists in the private sector, even among patients with similar insurance coverage).[60]

Increase Diversity in the Physician Workforce

Studies suggest that racial/ethnic concordance enhances physician-patient communication and that providers are less likely to recommend surgical care for black patients compared with white patients.[106,107] A recent analysis of surgical workforce diversity from 1996 to 2004 revealed an increase in the proportion of women in all 7 surgical specialties studied. In contrast, the proportion of black residents increased in only 4 surgical specialties and decreased in another 3. In addition, the proportion of black residents in every board-certified specialty workforce was lower than in the overall board-certified workforce during the study period. These studies underscore the importance of ongoing efforts by the American College of Surgeons to increase the number of racial/ethnic minorities entering surgical specialties.[108] Enhanced financial incentives (such as loan repayment programs) to qualified physicians who agree to practice in safety net hospitals that serve a disproportionate share of minority and underfunded patients should be strongly considered.

Expand Use of Patient Navigators

Patient navigation interventions are an evidence-based approach to reducing cancer disparities. Dr Harold P. Freeman created one of the first patient navigation programs in 1990 to help women in Harlem navigate the process of breast cancer screening and follow-up care.[109] Patient navigation is based on social support theory and is a barrier-focused intervention designed to ensure timely and efficient access to needed health services.[110–113] Navigators focus on case identification, identify psychosocial and practical barriers to care, and implement a care plan.[88,114]

Patient navigators can provide patients with information, in simple lay language, about treatment options and side effects, reduce misconceptions, and emphasize the importance of cancer treatments while acknowledging patients' fears and concerns. Patient navigators can develop trusted relationships with patients and help overcome potential mistrust of providers and the health care system.[53,115,116] Navigators can address economic barriers by connecting patients with resources and support systems, arranging for financial support, establishing reliable transportation, and assisting with out-of-pocket costs of care.[114,117,118] They can also contend with organizational and physician-patient communication barriers to cancer care by providing patients with patient-friendly informational materials about cancer and its treatment, coordinating care among multiple specialists, linking patients with appropriate follow-up care services, and reminding patient reminders about appointments.[109,113]

The NCI recently funded several sites to conduct and evaluate patient navigation interventions to promote cancer screening and treatment adherence.[119] In a subsequent review, the increased adherence to diagnostic follow-up care (after patient navigation) ranged from 21% to 29.2%.[109] In a randomized trial of navigation in a sample of low-income, ethnic minority women, the intervention group was more likely to be adherent through diagnostic resolution and to experience timely treatment than the usual care group.[120] In a patient navigation intervention to improve follow-up of abnormal breast cancer screening in an urban population, women in the intervention group had 39% greater odds of having timely follow-up.[114]

Expand Use of Active Comanagement

As discussed previously, the observed adverse effects of black race on postoperative outcomes after major cancer surgery may be partly explained by higher rates of underlying comorbidity at presentation and/or suboptimal structures or processes of care at the hospitals at which black and underfunded patients are treated.[22,24] Improved perioperative management of comorbid conditions could improve postoperative outcomes among blacks undergoing major surgery. This potentially can be achieved by increasing active co-management of cancer surgery patients by hospitalists experienced with perioperative care, particularly at hospitals caring for a disproportionate number of racial minorities and underinsured patients. Previous work suggests that hospitalist comanagement of orthopedic and cardiothoracic patients results in fewer complications, decreased mortality, and shortened lengths of stay.[121–124]

Increase Adherence to Best Practices

Third-party payers and regulatory agencies have begun focusing on National Quality Forum–endorsed, cancer-specific quality measures to reduce persistent variations in treatment across patient groups and communities. These measures are designed to enhance provider adherence to cancer-focused, best practice guidelines developed by organizations, such as the National Comprehensive Cancer Network and the American Society of Clinical Oncology. The American College of Surgeons Commission on Cancer has incorporated accountability and quality-improvement measures (centered around evidence-based adjuvant care for breast cancer, colon cancer, and rectal cancer) into the most current version of the Cancer Program Standards used to evaluate and rate institutions and programs seeking Commission on Cancer accreditation.[125] Programs participating in the Commission on Cancer Rapid Quality Reporting System can also track their performance with each of these measures in near real time and potentially intervene (at the patient level and/or provider level) when there is noncompliance with otherwise indicated cancer care.[126] To what extent these initiatives (and the eventual creation of cancer-specific pay-for-reporting and pay-for-performance process and outcome measures) may help reduce persistent racial disparities in cancer care and outcomes remains to be determined.

SUMMARY

The preponderance of the medical literature to date suggests that black-white differences in cancer outcomes are largely explained by failure to provide suitable cancer care rather than racial differences in stage at presentation, tumor biology, or response to treatments. Further studies using novel research methodologies and accounting for sociodemographic, physician, and hospital factors are needed to identify potentially modifiable patient and health care system factors that may underlie persistent racial disparities in receipt and quality of surgical and adjuvant therapy in patients with nonmetastatic breast cancer, lung cancer, and colorectal cancer. In the interim, ongoing efforts to improve access to care, enhance diversity in the surgical workforce, navigate minority cancer patients through the health care system, and enhance adherence to cancer-specific best practices are warranted.

REFERENCES

1. Siegel R, Ward E, Brawley O, et al. Cancer statistics, 2011: the impact of eliminating socioeconomic and racial disparities on premature cancer deaths. CA Cancer J Clin 2011;61(4):212–36.

2. Brawley OW. Disaggregating the effects of race and poverty on breast cancer outcomes. J Natl Cancer Inst 2002;94(7):471–3.
3. Chu KC, Tarone RE, Brawley OW. Breast cancer trends of black women compared with white women. Arch Fam Med 1999;8(6):521–8.
4. Chevarley F, White E. Recent trends in breast cancer mortality among white and black US women. Am J Public Health 1997;87(5):775–81.
5. Morris AM, Billingsley KG, Baxter NN, et al. Racial disparities in rectal cancer treatment: a population-based analysis. Arch Surg 2004;139(2):151–5 [discussion: 156].
6. Beart RW, Steele GD Jr, Menck HR, et al. Management and survival of patients with adenocarcinoma of the colon and rectum: a national survey of the Commission on Cancer. J Am Coll Surg 1995;181(3):225–36.
7. Jessup JM, McGinnis LS, Steele GD Jr, et al. The National Cancer Data Base. Report on colon cancer. Cancer 1996;78(4):918–26.
8. Villar HV, Menck HR. The National Cancer Data Base report on cancer in Hispanics. Relationships between ethnicity, poverty, and the diagnosis of some cancers. Cancer 1994;74(8):2386–95.
9. Mayberry RM, Coates RJ, Hill HA, et al. Determinants of black/white differences in colon cancer survival. J Natl Cancer Inst 1995;87(22):1686–93.
10. Bradley CJ, Given CW, Roberts C. Disparities in cancer diagnosis and survival. Cancer 2001;91(1):178–88.
11. Roetzheim RG, Pal N, Gonzalez EC, et al. Effects of health insurance and race on colorectal cancer treatments and outcomes. Am J Public Health 2000;90(11):1746–54.
12. Rogers SO, Ray WA, Smalley WE. A population-based study of survival among elderly persons diagnosed with colorectal cancer: does race matter if all are insured? (United States). Cancer Causes Control 2004;15(2):193–9.
13. Chen VW, Fenoglio-Preiser CM, Wu XC, et al. Aggressiveness of colon carcinoma in blacks and whites. National Cancer Institute Black/White Cancer Survival Study Group. Cancer Epidemiol Biomarkers Prev 1997;6(12):1087–93.
14. Esnaola NF, Stewart AK, Feig BW, et al. Age-, race-, and ethnicity-related differences in the treatment of nonmetastatic rectal cancer: a patterns of care study from the national cancer data base. Ann Surg Oncol 2008;15(11):3036–47.
15. Hegarty V, Burchett BM, Gold DT, et al. Racial differences in use of cancer prevention services among older Americans. J Am Geriatr Soc 2000;48(7):735–40.
16. Jatoi I, Anderson WF, Rao SR, et al. Breast cancer trends among black and white women in the United States. J Clin Oncol 2005;23(31):7836–41.
17. Dignam JJ, Colangelo L, Tian W, et al. Outcomes among African-Americans and Caucasians in colon cancer adjuvant therapy trials: findings from the National Surgical Adjuvant Breast and Bowel Project. J Natl Cancer Inst 1999;91(22):1933–40.
18. Dignam JJ, Ye Y, Colangelo L, et al. Prognosis after rectal cancer in blacks and whites participating in adjuvant therapy randomized trials. J Clin Oncol 2003;21(3):413–20.
19. Ball JK, Elixhauser A. Treatment differences between blacks and whites with colorectal cancer. Med Care 1996;34(9):970–84.
20. Bridges CR, Edwards FH, Peterson ED, et al. The effect of race on coronary bypass operative mortality. J Am Coll Cardiol 2000;36(6):1870–6.
21. Godley PA, Schenck AP, Amamoo MA, et al. Racial differences in mortality among Medicare recipients after treatment for localized prostate cancer. J Natl Cancer Inst 2003;95(22):1702–10.

22. Lucas FL, Stukel TA, Morris AM, et al. Race and surgical mortality in the United States. Ann Surg 2006;243(2):281–6.

23. Nathan H, Frederick W, Choti MA, et al. Racial disparity in surgical mortality after major hepatectomy. J Am Coll Surg 2008;207(3):312–9.

24. Esnaola NF, Hall BL, Hosokawa PW, et al. Race and surgical outcomes: it is not all black and white. Ann Surg 2008;248(4):647–55.

25. Charlson ME, Pompei P, Ales KL, et al. A new method of classifying prognostic comorbidity in longitudinal studies: development and validation. J Chronic Dis 1987;40(5):373–83.

26. Kimmick G, Muss HB, Case LD, et al. A comparison of treatment outcomes for black patients and white patients with metastatic breast cancer. The Piedmont Oncology Association experience. Cancer 1991;67(11):2850–4.

27. Roach M 3rd, Cirrincione C, Budman D, et al. Race and survival from breast cancer: based on Cancer and Leukemia Group B trial 8541. Cancer J Sci Am 1997;3(2):107–12.

28. Dignam JJ, Redmond CK, Fisher B, et al. Prognosis among African-American women and white women with lymph node negative breast carcinoma: findings from two randomized clinical trials of the National Surgical Adjuvant Breast and Bowel Project (NSABP). Cancer 1997;80(1):80–90.

29. Du W, Simon MS. Racial disparities in treatment and survival of women with stage I-III breast cancer at a large academic medical center in metropolitan Detroit. Breast Cancer Res Treat 2005;91:243–8.

30. Connor CS, Touijer AK, Krishnan L, et al. Local recurrence following breast conservation therapy in African-American women with invasive breast cancer. Am J Surg 2000;179(1):22–6.

31. Dignam JJ. Efficacy of systemic adjuvant therapy for breast cancer in African-American and Caucasian women. J Natl Cancer Inst Monogr 2001;(30):36–43.

32. Bach PB, Cramer LD, Warren JL, et al. Racial differences in the treatment of early-stage lung cancer. N Engl J Med 1999;341(16):1198–205.

33. Lathan CS, Neville BA, Earle CC. The effect of race on invasive staging and surgery in non-small-cell lung cancer. J Clin Oncol 2006;24(3):413–8.

34. Graham MV, Geitz LM, Byhardt R, et al. Comparison of prognostic factors and survival among black patients and white patients treated with irradiation for non-small-cell lung cancer. J Natl Cancer Inst 1992;84(22):1731–5.

35. Akerley WL 3rd, Moritz TE, Ryan LS, et al. Racial comparison of outcomes of male Department of Veterans Affairs patients with lung and colon cancer. Arch Intern Med 1993;153(14):1681–8.

36. Shavers VL, Brown ML. Racial and ethnic disparities in the receipt of cancer treatment. J Natl Cancer Inst 2002;94(5):334–57.

37. Muss HB, Hunter CP, Wesley M, et al. Treatment plans for black and white women with stage II node-positive breast cancer. The National Cancer Institute Black/White Cancer Survival Study experience. Cancer 1992;70(10):2460–7.

38. Heimann R, Ferguson D, Powers C, et al. Race and clinical outcome in breast cancer in a series with long-term follow-up evaluation. J Clin Oncol 1997;15(6):2329–37.

39. Michalski TA, Nattinger AB. The influence of black race and socioeconomic status on the use of breast-conserving surgery for Medicare beneficiaries. Cancer 1997;79(2):314–9.

40. Velanovich V, Yood MU, Bawle U, et al. Racial differences in the presentation and surgical management of breast cancer. Surgery 1999;125(4):375–9.

41. Bradley CJ, Given CW, Roberts C. Race, socioeconomic status, and breast cancer treatment and survival. J Natl Cancer Inst 2002;94(7):490–6.
42. Esnaola NF, Knott K, Finney C, et al. Urban/rural residence moderates effect of race on receipt of surgery in patients with nonmetastatic breast cancer: a report from the South Carolina central cancer registry. Ann Surg Oncol 2008;15(7): 1828–36.
43. Lin AY, Ihde DC. Recent developments in the treatment of lung cancer. JAMA 1992;267(12):1661–4.
44. Greenwald HP, Polissar NL, Borgatta EF, et al. Social factors, treatment, and survival in early-stage non-small cell lung cancer. Am J Public Health 1998; 88(11):1681–4.
45. Esnaola NF, Gebregziabher M, Knott K, et al. Underuse of surgical resection for localized, non-small cell lung cancer among whites and African Americans in South Carolina. Ann Thorac Surg 2008;86(1):220–6 [discussion: 227].
46. Cooper GS, Yuan Z, Landefeld CS, et al. Surgery for colorectal cancer: race-related differences in rates and survival among Medicare beneficiaries. Am J Public Health 1996;86(4):582–6.
47. Esnaola NF, Gebregziabher M, Finney C, et al. Underuse of surgical resection in black patients with nonmetastatic colorectal cancer: location, location, location. Ann Surg 2009;250(4):549–57.
48. Bickell NA, Wang JJ, Oluwole S, et al. Missed opportunities: racial disparities in adjuvant breast cancer treatment. J Clin Oncol 2006;24(9):1357–62.
49. Ballard-Barbash R, Potosky AL, Harlan LC, et al. Factors associated with surgical and radiation therapy for early stage breast cancer in older women. J Natl Cancer Inst 1996;88(11):716–26.
50. Riley GF, Potosky AL, Klabunde CN, et al. Stage at diagnosis and treatment patterns among older women with breast cancer: an HMO and fee-for-service comparison. JAMA 1999;281(8):720–6.
51. Schrag D, Gelfand SE, Bach PB, et al. Who gets adjuvant treatment for stage II and III rectal cancer? Insight from surveillance, epidemiology, and end results—Medicare. J Clin Oncol 2001;19(17):3712–8.
52. McGory ML, Zingmond DS, Sekeris E, et al. A patient's race/ethnicity does not explain the underuse of appropriate adjuvant therapy in colorectal cancer. Dis Colon Rectum 2006;49(3):319–29.
53. Gansler T, Henley SJ, Stein K, et al. Sociodemographic determinants of cancer treatment health literacy. Cancer 2005;104(3):653–60.
54. Margolis ML, Christie JD, Silvestri GA, et al. Racial differences pertaining to a belief about lung cancer surgery: results of a multicenter survey. Ann Intern Med 2003;139(7):558–63.
55. Cykert S, Dilworth-Anderson P, Monroe MH, et al. Factors associated with decisions to undergo surgery among patients with newly diagnosed early-stage lung cancer. JAMA 2010;303(23):2368–76.
56. McNeil BJ, Weichselbaum R, Pauker SG. Speech and survival: tradeoffs between quality and quantity of life in laryngeal cancer. N Engl J Med 1981; 305(17):982–7.
57. Oddone EZ, Horner RD, Johnston DC, et al. Carotid endarterectomy and race: do clinical indications and patient preferences account for differences? Stroke 2002;33(12):2936–43.
58. Bosworth HB, Stechuchak KM, Grambow SC, et al. Patient risk perceptions for carotid endarterectomy: which patients are strongly averse to surgery? J Vasc Surg 2004;40(1):86–91.

59. Demissie K, Oluwole OO, Balasubramanian BA, et al. Racial differences in the treatment of colorectal cancer: a comparison of surgical and radiation therapy between Whites and Blacks. Ann Epidemiol 2004;14(3):215–21.
60. Bach PB, Pham HH, Schrag D, et al. Primary care physicians who treat blacks and whites. N Engl J Med 2004;351(6):575–84.
61. Dominitz JA, Samsa GP, Landsman P, et al. Race, treatment, and survival among colorectal carcinoma patients in an equal-access medical system. Cancer 1998;82(12):2312–20.
62. McCann J, Artinian V, Duhaime L, et al. Evaluation of the causes for racial disparity in surgical treatment of early stage lung cancer. Chest 2005;128(5): 3440–6.
63. Silvestri GA, Knittig S, Zoller JS, et al. Importance of faith on medical decisions regarding cancer care. J Clin Oncol 2003;21(7):1379–82.
64. Levinson W, Hudak PL, Feldman JJ, et al. "It's not what you say.": racial disparities in communication between orthopedic surgeons and patients. Med Care 2008;46(4):410–6.
65. Jessup JM, Stewart A, Greene FL, et al. Adjuvant chemotherapy for stage III colon cancer: implications of race/ethnicity, age, and differentiation. JAMA 2005;294(21):2703–11.
66. van Ryn M, Burke J. The effect of patient race and socio-economic status on physicians' perceptions of patients. Soc Sci Med 2000;50(6):813–28.
67. Mandelblatt JS, Kerner JF, Hadley J, et al. Variations in breast carcinoma treatment in older medicare beneficiaries: is it black or white. Cancer 2002;95(7): 1401–14.
68. Silvestri GA, Handy J, Lackland D, et al. Specialists achieve better outcomes than generalists for lung cancer surgery. Chest 1998;114(3):675–80.
69. Schrag D, Panageas KS, Riedel E, et al. Hospital and surgeon procedure volume as predictors of outcome following rectal cancer resection. Ann Surg 2002;236(5):583–92.
70. Nattinger AB, Gottlieb MS, Veum J, et al. Geographic variation in the use of breast-conserving treatment for breast cancer. N Engl J Med 1992;326(17): 1102–7.
71. Liu JH, Zingmond DS, McGory ML, et al. Disparities in the utilization of high-volume hospitals for complex surgery. JAMA 2006;296(16):1973–80.
72. Neighbors CJ, Rogers ML, Shenassa ED, et al. Ethnic/racial disparities in hospital procedure volume for lung resection for lung cancer. Med Care 2007; 45(7):655–63.
73. Khuri SF, Daley J, Henderson W, et al. Relation of surgical volume to outcome in eight common operations: results from the VA National Surgical Quality Improvement Program. Ann Surg 1999;230(3):414–29 [discussion: 429–32].
74. Birkmeyer JD. High-risk surgery–follow the crowd. JAMA 2000;283(9):1191–3.
75. Gill T, Taylor AW, Pengelly A. A population-based survey of factors relating to the prevalence of falls in older people. Gerontology 2005;51(5):340–5.
76. Birkmeyer JD, Dimick JB. Potential benefits of the new Leapfrog standards: effect of process and outcomes measures. Surgery 2004;135(6):569–75.
77. Ward MM, Jaana M, Wakefield DS, et al. What would be the effect of referral to high-volume hospitals in a largely rural state? J Rural Health 2004;20(4):344–54.
78. Meyerhardt JA, Tepper JE, Niedzwiecki D, et al. Impact of hospital procedure volume on surgical operation and long-term outcomes in high-risk curatively resected rectal cancer: findings from the Intergroup 0114 Study. J Clin Oncol 2004;22(1):166–74.

79. Breslin TM, Morris AM, Gu N, et al. Hospital factors and racial disparities in mortality after surgery for breast and colon cancer. J Clin Oncol 2009;27(24): 3945–50.
80. Rhoads KF, Ackerson LK, Jha AK, et al. Quality of colon cancer outcomes in hospitals with a high percentage of Medicaid patients. J Am Coll Surg 2008; 207(2):197–204.
81. Onega T, Duell EJ, Shi X, et al. Race versus place of service in mortality among medicare beneficiaries with cancer. Cancer 2010;116(11):2698–706.
82. Egede LE. Race, ethnicity, culture, and disparities in health care. J Gen Intern Med 2006;21(6):667–9.
83. Cooper R, David R. The biological concept of race and its application to public health and epidemiology. J Health Polit Policy Law 1986;11(1):97–116.
84. Williams DR. The concept of race in Health Services Research: 1966 to 1990. Health Serv Res 1994;29(3):261–74.
85. Dunmore C, Plummer P, Regan G, et al. Re: race and differences in breast cancer survival in a managed care population. J Natl Cancer Inst 2000;92(20):1690–1.
86. Tropman SE, Ricketts TC, Paskett E, et al. Rural breast cancer treatment: evidence from the Reaching Communities for Cancer Care (REACH) project. Breast Cancer Res Treat 1999;56(1):59–66.
87. Bryant H, Mah Z. Breast cancer screening attitudes and behaviors of rural and urban women. Prev Med 1992;21(4):405–18.
88. Doll R, Stephen J, Barroetavena MC, et al. Patient navigation in cancer care: final report. Vancouver, British Columbia, Canada: Sociobehavioural Research Centre BC Cancer Agency; 2005.
89. Fletcher C, Flora J, Gaddis B, et al. Small towns and welfare reform: Iowa case studies of families and communities. Paper presented at: Rural Dimensions of Welfare Reform: A Research Conference on Poverty, Welfare, and Food Assistance 2000, Georgetown University. Washington, DC, May 4–5, 2010.
90. Schur C, Franco SJ. Access to health care. Rural health in the United States. New York: Oxford University Press; 1999.
91. Fernandez ME, Gonzales A, Tortolero-Luna G, et al. Using intervention mapping to develop a breast and cervical cancer screening program for Hispanic farmworkers: Cultivando La Salud. Health Promot Pract 2005;6(4):394–404.
92. Morris AM, Rhoads KF, Stain SC, et al. Understanding racial disparities in cancer treatment and outcomes. J Am Coll Surg 2010;211(1):105–13.
93. Statements of the American College of Surgeons: Statement on Health Care Disparities. 2001. Available at: http://www.facs.org/fellows_info/statements/st-67.html. Accessed September 15, 2011.
94. Greenwald HP, Polissar NL, Borgatta EF, et al. Detecting survival effects of socioeconomic status: problems in the use of aggregate measures. J Clin Epidemiol 1994;47(8):903–9.
95. Deyo RA, Cherkin DC, Ciol MA. Adapting a clinical comorbidity index for use with ICD-9-CM administrative databases. J Clin Epidemiol 1992;45(6):613–9.
96. Romano PS, Roos LL, Jollis JG. Adapting a clinical comorbidity index for use with ICD-9-CM administrative data: differing perspectives. J Clin Epidemiol 1993;46(10):1075–9 [discussion: 1081–90].
97. Slee VN. The International Classification of Diseases: ninth revision (ICD-9). Ann Intern Med 1978;88(3):424–6.
98. Hsia DC, Krushat WM, Fagan AB, et al. Accuracy of diagnostic coding for Medicare patients under the prospective-payment system. N Engl J Med 1988; 318(6):352–5.

99. Khuri SF, Daley J, Henderson W, et al. The National Veterans Administration Surgical Risk Study: risk adjustment for the comparative assessment of the quality of surgical care. J Am Coll Surg 1995;180(5):519–31.

100. Khuri SF, Daley J, Henderson W, et al. The Department of Veterans Affairs' NSQIP: the first national, validated, outcome-based, risk-adjusted, and peer-controlled program for the measurement and enhancement of the quality of surgical care. National VA Surgical Quality Improvement Program. Ann Surg 1998;228(4):491–507.

101. Atherly A, Fink AS, Campbell DC, et al. Evaluating alternative risk-adjustment strategies for surgery. Am J Surg 2004;188(5):566–70.

102. Begg CB, Cramer LD, Hoskins WJ, et al. Impact of hospital volume on operative mortality for major cancer surgery. JAMA 1998;280(20):1747–51.

103. Birkmeyer JD, Siewers AE, Finlayson EV, et al. Hospital volume and surgical mortality in the United States. N Engl J Med 2002;346(15):1128–37.

104. Birkmeyer JD, Stukel TA, Siewers AE, et al. Surgeon volume and operative mortality in the United States. N Engl J Med 2003;349(22):2117–27.

105. Viswanathan M, Nerz P, Dalberth B, et al. Assessing the Impact of AHRQ Evidence-Based Practice Center (EPC) Reports on Future Research. Rockville (MD): Agency for Healthcare Research and Quality (US); 2011.

106. Johnson RL, Roter D, Powe NR, et al. Patient race/ethnicity and quality of patient-physician communication during medical visits. Am J Public Health 2004;94(12):2084–90.

107. Cooper-Patrick L, Gallo JJ, Gonzales JJ, et al. Race, gender, and partnership in the patient-physician relationship. JAMA 1999;282(6):583–9.

108. Statements of the American College of Surgeons: Statement on Diversity. 2001. Available at: http://www.facs.org/fellows_info/statements/st-37.html. Accessed September 15, 2011.

109. Wells KJ, Battaglia TA, Dudley DJ, et al. Patient navigation: state of the art or is it science? Cancer 2008;113(8):1999–2010.

110. Bradford JB, Coleman S, Cunningham W. HIV System Navigation: an emerging model to improve HIV care access. AIDS Patient Care STDS 2007;21(Suppl 1):S49–58.

111. Dohan D, Schrag D. Using navigators to improve care of underserved patients: current practices and approaches. Cancer 2005;104(4):848–55.

112. Psooy BJ, Schreuer D, Borgaonkar J, et al. Patient navigation: improving timeliness in the diagnosis of breast abnormalities. Can Assoc Radiol J 2004;55(3):145–50.

113. Vargas RB, Ryan GW, Jackson CA, et al. Characteristics of the original patient navigation programs to reduce disparities in the diagnosis and treatment of breast cancer. Cancer 2008;113(2):426–33.

114. Battaglia TA, Roloff K, Posner MA, et al. Improving follow-up to abnormal breast cancer screening in an urban population. A patient navigation intervention. Cancer 2007;109(Suppl 2):359–67.

115. Gerend MA, Pai M. Social determinants of Black-White disparities in breast cancer mortality: a review. Cancer Epidemiol Biomarkers Prev 2008;17(11):2913–23.

116. Doll R, Stephens J, Barroetavena M, et al. Patient navigation in cancer care: final report. Vancouver (British Columbia): Sociobehavioural Research Centre; 2003.

117. Freeman HP, Muth BJ, Kerner JF. Expanding access to cancer screening and clinical follow-up among the medically underserved. Cancer Pract 1995;3(1):19–30.

118. Fillion L, de Serres M, Lapointe-Goupil R, et al. Implementing the role of patient-navigator nurse at a university hospital centre. Can Oncol Nurs J 2006;16(1): 11–7, 5–10.
119. Freund KM, Battaglia TA, Calhoun E, et al. National Cancer Institute Patient Navigation Research Program: methods, protocol, and measures. Cancer 2008; 113(12):3391–9.
120. Ell K, Vourlekis B, Lee PJ, et al. Patient navigation and case management following an abnormal mammogram: a randomized clinical trial. Prev Med 2007;44(1):26–33.
121. Phy MP, Vanness DJ, Melton LJ 3rd, et al. Effects of a hospitalist model on elderly patients with hip fracture. Arch Intern Med 2005;165(7):796–801.
122. Huddleston JM, Long KH, Naessens JM, et al. Medical and surgical comanagement after elective hip and knee arthroplasty: a randomized, controlled trial. Ann Intern Med 2004;141(1):28–38.
123. Fisher AA, Davis MW, Rubenach SE, et al. Outcomes for older patients with hip fractures: the impact of orthopedic and geriatric medicine cocare. J Orthop Trauma 2006;20(3):172–8 [discussion: 179–80].
124. Macpherson DS, Parenti C, Nee J, et al. An internist joins the surgery service: does comanagement make a difference? J Gen Intern Med 1994;9(8):440–4.
125. Cancer Program Standards 2012: Ensuring Patient-Centered Care. 2011. Available at: http://www.facs.org/cancer/coc/programstandards2012.html. Accessed October 15, 2011.
126. Rapid Quality Reporting System (RQRS). 2011. Available at: http://www.facs.org/cancer/ncdb/rqrs.html. Accessed October 15, 2011.

Prediction Tools in Surgical Oncology

Brandon K. Isariyawongse, MD[a], Michael W. Kattan, PhD[b],*

KEYWORDS

- Nomograms • Oncology • Outcomes • Predictive models

KEY POINTS

- The contemporary patient is a savvy consumer of medical goods and services with information requirements that typically extend beyond that which is provided by physicians limited by the demands of modern-day clinic schedules.
- Prediction tools function to replicate the critical synthesization of data regularly conducted by physicians in a succinct, reproducible, unbiased, and evidence-based format that can be seamlessly incorporated into the patient visit.
- Current models have been shown to accurately predict a wide variety of oncologic outcomes, but there is an emerging need for the development of prediction tools that address quality of life end points.
- The incorporation of multiple validated prediction models into comparative effectiveness tables, which provide a side-by-side comparison of medical options with respect to the expected benefits and harms of therapy, can provide patients with the high-quality informed consent that they require to make a fully informed treatment decision.

INTRODUCTION

Now more than ever, patients who receive a diagnosis of cancer have the potential to be overwhelmed with the abundance of decisions presented to them for oncologic therapy. Long gone are the times when the therapeutic options were limited simply to such alternatives as surgery or chemotherapy. Rather, with the advent of novel chemotherapeutic regimens, intensity-modulated radiation therapy protocols, and advances in surgical technique, particularly with the evolution of minimally invasive approaches, the oncologic patient might be presented with choices A through G as opposed to merely A and B. As the number of available therapeutic options expands, the amount of diagnostic and prognostic information that is pertinent to the patient grows concurrently.

Dr Kattan is a consultant for Dendreon and Sanofi-Aventis.
[a] Department of Urology, Glickman Urological and Kidney Institute, Cleveland Clinic Foundation, 9500 Euclid Avenue/Q-10, Cleveland, OH 44195, USA; [b] Department of Quantitative and Health Sciences, Cleveland Clinic Foundation, 9500 Euclid Avenue/JJN3-01, Cleveland, OH 44195, USA
* Corresponding author.
E-mail address: kattanm@ccf.org

The contemporary patient is a savvy consumer of medical goods and services, and patients are no longer approaching medical visits ready to take notes with a blank sheet of paper. Quite the opposite, the modern visit to the physician's office is often accompanied by knowledge gathered from the anecdotal information of friends and family, in addition to the overabundance of information available by way of a basic Internet connection. On-line forums allow a patient to connect with others with similar diagnoses who, previously worlds apart, now are united by a few simple keystrokes.[1] Although these facts and figures (sometimes valid, oftentimes not) are considered invaluable to the patient with cancer teeming with anxiety and angst over a new diagnosis, the burden falls on the physician to sift through this newfound information and provide an accurate and unbiased representation of prognosis, diagnosis, and therapy. It is this critical synthesization of data that patients rely on most when making treatment decisions.

Unfortunately, despite the wide range of information provided to patients, the evidence demonstrates that physicians often fall short of meeting the information needs and expectations of patients.[2,3] There is widespread recognition that patients who are better-informed before therapy experience improved psychosocial outcomes after therapy.[4,5] Several studies have indicated that patients would prefer to receive even more information and physician guidance than is generally presented to them, and accurate estimates of the likelihood of treatment success, complications, and morbidity are critical to patients seeking to make fully informed treatment decisions.[6,7] However, in the current state of medicine, the limitations placed on physicians with crowded clinic schedules and constrained counseling time are not minor, and appropriately navigating the landscape of limited time with increased expectations requires that physicians maximize efficiency and at the same time adequately address the concerns of the patient.

ARTIFICIAL NEURAL NETWORKS, PREDICTION TABLES, AND NOMOGRAMS

Conventionally, risk estimations and outcomes prognosis have been based primarily on physician judgment. However, physician estimations are inherently fraught with unintentional and intentional bias, and interest has grown in the development of prediction tools that can provide patients with a concise and balanced representation of their diagnostic and prognostic outcomes.[8–10] Many of these instruments have developed into "bedside" tools that can be used expeditiously and provide patients with information in an easily digestible format.[11] Examples of prediction tools that have been popularized include artificial neural networks (ANN), probability tables, and nomograms.

ANN are computer-generated algorithms that function to assimilate information in the same way that a brain does in response to various inputs. Although the algorithmic generation of the ANN is beyond the scope of this article, generally the ANN is comprised of several layers of information, and these layers, which consist of discrete neurons or knots, are bound together by various links along with signals travel. The output generated depends on the various inputs received from the input layers and has the advantage of incorporating multiple complex variable relationships. The ANN model has been used in areas of oncology including breast, gastric, and prostate cancer for diagnosis and prognosis but has been largely supplanted by nomograms and prediction tables because of the latter's improved accuracy and ease of incorporation into modern medical practice.[12–14]

Prediction tables have the benefit of providing outcome measures in an easily interpretable format that can be presented and applied to any patient in clinic. Typically, the prediction tables incorporate relevant pretreatment variables and provide individualized risk estimates based on the variables that each patient brings to the table. This theory of individualized medicine (outcomes based on a patient's personal clinicopathologic parameters) is immensely more attractive than receiving an overarching percentage chance of cure based on a clinical trial comprised of patients with widely varied disease states. One of the primary drawbacks of prediction tables lies in their inherent inability to keep variables that are continuous in clinical practice (eg, serum prostate-specific antigen [PSA]) continuous in the model. By categorizing those continuous variables and placing them into discrete boxes, one assumes that risk is constant within groups and increases sharply at categorical boundaries, and in the process, part of the intrinsic predictive value of the variable is wasted. This is a shortcoming that is not shared with nomograms, and several studies have identified an advantage in predictive accuracy in nomograms compared with prediction tables.[15,16]

Nomograms are a graphical representation of a mathematical formula. Regardless of the statistical methods used (most often multivariate logistic regression or Cox proportional hazards analysis) the development of a nomogram includes multiple clinical parameters, which may be either continuous or categorical, each of which is represented by a scale based on its statistical impact on the specified outcome. The scales for each statistically significant predictive variable are then plotted in a visual format such that each corresponds to a numerical value; the tally of these values among all variables can then be converted into the probability of reaching the outcome. The use of nomograms in clinical practice offers the advantage of condensing a complicated mathematical formula into a simple and easily interpretable format and one that can be applied efficiently at the time of a patient visit, thereby providing a wealth of information in a short period of time. The nomogram essentially functions to replicate the synthesization of data the physicians conduct on a daily basis in a reproducible, unbiased, and evidence-based format that can be seamlessly incorporated into each patient visit. Furthermore, although nomograms function to reproduce clinical judgment, their predictive value has been shown to outperform the predictions of clinicians in some circumstances.[17–19]

EXAMPLES OF CLINICAL PREDICTION TOOLS
Predicting Pathologic Stage in Prostate Cancer

Although most men diagnosed with prostate cancer have clinically organ-confined disease (clinical stage T2 or less), some evidence suggests that more than 50% of patients who go on to radical prostatectomy have pathologic evidence of extraprostatic spread of the disease and thus may require multimodal therapy for any chance of cure.[20] Partin and colleagues[21–23] devised a series of tables based on clinical T stage, serum PSA, and grade of prostatic adenocarcinoma by transrectal ultrasound-guided biopsy that provides percentage estimates of pathologic stage, including organ-confined disease, extracapsular extension, and invasion of the seminal vesicles to help guide treatment decisions; the tables have since been updated to reflect more contemporary clinicopathologic data. These tables have come to be known as the "Partin tables," and were one of the first ubiquitous prediction models in prostate cancer, which has now experienced a surge in the number of available prediction tools.

Nomogram Predicting Malignancy in Thyroid Nodules

With the continual progress of radiologic techniques, an increasing number of subclinical thyroid nodules are being detected. The appropriate management of these nodules is controversial, because only a small percentage are truly malignant and the limitations of an often nondiagnostic percutaneous fine-needle aspiration are well-recognized.[24] Thus, preemptive surgical excision likely overtreats most nodules, whereas a protocol of observation until the appearance of more definitive signs of malignancy delays curative treatment for an unpredictable period of time. To tackle this clinical dilemma, Nixon and colleagues[25] developed a nomogram based on clinical, biochemical, radiologic, and pathologic features to predict the risk of malignancy in thyroid nodules. Although the counseling physician certainly could take the time to explain the relevance of thyroid-stimulating hormone levels, nodule echo-texture, and nodule vascularity and how those variables affect risk of malignancy, the clinical nomogram provides a visual representation from which patients can see with their own eyes what factors have the most bearing on the outcome of interest. Additionally, patients can be reassured that the nomogram produces a result that is individualized based on his or her clinicopathologic parameters and does not contain anecdotal bias.

Preoperative and Postoperative Nomograms Predicting Disease Recurrence after Radical Prostatectomy

In terms of cancer screening and posttherapeutic surveillance, the advent of the PSA era has permanently transformed the field of urologic oncology. By increasing the lead time diagnosis of prostate cancer, there has been an expected decline in the average age at diagnosis for the disease worldwide, and an increasing number of men are surviving multiple decades as opposed to multiple years after radical prostatectomy in what has historically been a disease of older men.[26,27] With PSA now serving as the primary mode of postprostatectomy surveillance, a rising PSA after definitive therapy has emerged as a new end point for oncologic recurrence before symptomatic disease and has been termed "biochemical recurrence." Seeking to characterize postoperative outcomes before radical prostatectomy, our group first developed a nomogram predicting a patient's preoperative risk of biochemical recurrence based on tumor grade, PSA level, and clinical stage.[28] The nomogram has since been updated to include other preoperative variables, such as biopsy cores positive for cancer, and a postoperative version has also been developed to further aid in patient counseling (**Fig. 1**).[29,30] Thus, this predictive model provides patients with critical information

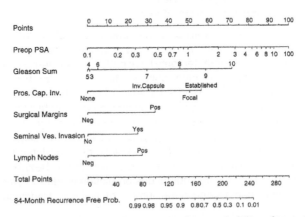

Fig. 1. Nomogram predicting 84-month recurrence-free probability after radical prostatectomy for adenocarcinoma of the prostate based on preoperative and postoperative clinicopathologic variables. A straight line drawn from each variable to the point's axis at the top of the nomogram determines how many points toward recurrence the patient receives. A sum of the points for each variable based on the total point's axis at the bottom of the nomogram corresponds to the predicted recurrence-free probability. (*From* Kattan MW, Wheeler TM, Scardino PT. Postoperative nomogram for disease recurrence after radical prostatectomy for prostate cancer. J Clin Oncol 1999;17(5):1499–507; with permission.)

regarding prognostic outcomes after definitive therapy for adenocarcinoma of the prostate with performance that has been validated externally in multiple patient cohorts.[31,32]

Benefit of Adjuvant Chemotherapy in Patients with Colon Cancer

Although there is widespread agreement that fluorouracil-based therapy benefits patients with advanced colon cancer, it is not clear which subgroups of patients benefit the most from adjuvant chemotherapy. To tackle this clinical question, Gill and colleagues[33] performed a pooled analysis and created a table that predicts overall and disease-free survival stratified by age, nodal status, and tumor grade and T stage. In this way, the patient may make an informed postoperative decision based on his or her own calculated benefit weighed against treatment-related toxicity. The authors of this study have used the results of their work to create an on-line clinical calculator, which is available at http://www.mayoclinic.com/calcs and permits widespread public use of their data.

EVALUATING AND COMPARING PREDICTION TOOLS

The recent expansion in the armamentarium of prediction tools, although encouraging from an evidence-based medicine standpoint, has created a new challenge in the form of evaluating models for quality and applicability and, furthermore, determining which prediction tool to use in the case of similar models.

After settling on an established, relevant end point predicted by the model, our recommendation is first to ensure that the model was based on a population that is demographically and temporally similar to the patient population to whom the tool is being applied. Just as we are cautious to apply the outcomes of clinical work from different countries or time periods, one must always be cognizant of the population demographics and time period for patient accrual, which if significantly different may significantly weaken the applicability of the model. In general, prediction tools derived from larger datasets provide more robust results, with the caveat that large gaps in records (ie, missing values) tend to suggest systematic issues with the data (**Box 1**). Those models that contain all available prognostic variables, although somewhat limited in practicality, generally have an advantage in predictive accuracy. When generating the model itself, stepwise variable selection tends to produce less accurate prediction tools; we advocate using tools that model fit statistics throughout the entire model-building process, as opposed to selecting out variables based on P values arising from univariate analyses. Be wary of nomograms that categorize continuous variables, because one of the primary benefits of nomograms is the ability to keep

---

Box 1
Properties of good prediction tools

- Large sample size
- Includes all routinely available predictors
- No univariable screening
- Continuous variables are kept continuous
- Nonlinear effects are allowed
- Few missing values in dataset
- Close to 45-degree calibration curve

Table 1 Comparative effectiveness	Treatment X	Treatment Y
Benefits		
Benefit 1	B1%	B1%
Benefit 2	B2%	B2%
Harms		
Harm 1	H1%	H1%
Harm 2	H2%	H2%

Each cell is populated by means of individualized predictions by existing models based on either treatment choice X or treatment choice Y.

variables that are continuous in clinical practice continuous in the model. Furthermore, a nomogram that permits variables to have nonlinear effects is better than one that does not. Objectively, the concordance index, which gives the probability that for a randomly selected pair of patients the model will assign a higher probability to the patient who had the event, ranges from 0.5 to 1 and can be useful in comparing prediction tools but ideally is interpreted only in the setting of neutral data to eliminate any confounders.

FUTURE OF PREDICTION TOOLS

The popularity of prediction tools, such as nomograms, has led to more than a surplus of available models, with many more on the horizon that are in the process of development. However, despite this influx of models into the oncologic literature, there is a lack of head-to-head model comparisons and also insufficient external validation of currently published tools. To be fair, most published models are validated internally on the same data on which they were generated, but external validation provides evidence for broad applicability of the prediction tool by means of an independent dataset. Rather than producing a new tool and moving forward with the creation of a new model, it is prudent first to validate the initial tool on an independent dataset to complete the work and firmly establish its contribution to the current literature.

Although the bulk of clinical prediction tools have focused on oncologic outcome, predictions for quality of life outcomes have been much less common in the literature. With the excess of information at their disposal, modern patients are well aware of the morbidity associated with cancer therapies, and some patients may choose to forego therapy to avoid treatment-related side effects if the risk is substantial. This has become no more apparent than in the field of prostate cancer, where more and more patients with low-risk disease are electing to postpone definitive treatment and instead follow an active surveillance protocol to delay, and possibly avoid altogether, the treatment-related side effects of radical prostatectomy or radiation therapy, which include erectile dysfunction, urinary incontinence, and bowel and bladder dysfunction.[34] Even when making decisions between therapies, active surveillance notwithstanding, patients may prefer to weigh morbidity risks in concert with oncologic risks, and prediction tools that can provide these approximations up-front would arm them with the information that they need to make a well-informed treatment decision. Given the contemporary emphasis on the minimization of treatment-related morbidity, it is clear that there is opportunity to produce newer predictive models that would address this gap in the literature, although this is dependent on available and reliable quality of life data, which may or may not be appropriately mature at this time.

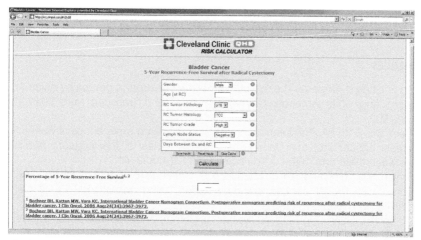

Fig. 2. An example of an on-line clinical risk calculator predicting 5-year recurrence-free survival after radical cystectomy for bladder cancer. This calculator, along with others, is available at http://rcalc.ccf.org. RC, radical cystectomy.

Provided what is known about the information needs of patients, the goal should be to supply the patient with an individualized risk assessment based on validated prediction models that addresses not only oncologic outcomes but also morbidity associated with therapy. This will enable patients to derive the maximum predictive benefit from their own specific clinicopathologic variables. A side-by-side comparison of medical options with respect to the expected benefits and expected harms would allow a patient to make an informed and individualized treatment decision based on the outcomes that he or she values most; this type of comparison is termed "comparative effectiveness." By combining prediction tools that address morbidity and mortality, a thorough pretreatment comparative effectiveness table (**Table 1**) can be generated that can serve as high-quality informed consent for the patient struggling with the treatment decision.[35] Some of the limiting factors in generating a thorough comparative effectiveness table are the availability of sufficient quality of life nomograms and predictive models that have been independently validated for application across patient populations. Although some may argue that making multiple predictions during an office visit may be burdensome or time-consuming, such Web sites as http://www.nomograms.org and http://rcalc.ccf.org have demonstrated that simple, accurate, and informative predictions are but a few button-clicks away (**Fig. 2**).

SUMMARY

In the era of severely limited physician clinic time yet increased patient information needs and expectations, the modern office visit must become a model of efficiency by means of succinct but informative counsel. Prediction tools, such as ANN, prediction tables, and clinical nomograms, afford physicians the ability to transmit an immense amount of prognostic information in a format that exhibits as much comprehensibility as it does brevity. Current models demonstrate that it is feasible to accurately predict a wide array of oncologic outcomes, including pathologic stage, recurrence-free survival, and response to adjuvant therapy. Although emphasis should be placed on the independent validation of existing prediction tools, there is a paucity of models in the literature that focus on quality of life outcomes. Ultimately, the unification of tools that predict oncologic and quality of life outcomes into a comparative effectiveness table will furnish cancer patients with the information they need to make a highly informed and individualized treatment decision.

REFERENCES

1. Im EO, Lee B, Chee W. The use of Internet cancer support groups by Asian Americans and white Americans living with cancer. J Transcult Nurs 2011;22(4): 386–96.
2. Rees CE, Bath PA. The information needs and source preferences of women with breast cancer and their family members: a review of the literature published between 1988 and 1998. J Adv Nurs 2000;31(4):833–41.
3. Smyth MM, McCaughan E, Harrisson S. Women's perceptions of their experiences with breast cancer: are their needs being addressed? Eur J Cancer Care (Engl) 1995;4(2):86–92.
4. Butow PN, Dunn SM, Tattersall MH, et al. Computer-based interaction analysis of the cancer consultation. Br J Cancer 1995;71(5):1115–21.
5. Rainey LC. Effects of preparatory patient education for radiation oncology patients. Cancer 1985;56(5):1056–61.
6. Cassileth BR, Zupkis RV, Sutton-Smith K, et al. Information and participation preferences among cancer patients. Ann Intern Med 1980;92(6):832–6.
7. Jenkins V, Fallowfield L, Saul J. Information needs of patients with cancer: results from a large study in UK cancer centres. Br J Cancer 2001;84(1):48–51.
8. Fowler FJ Jr, McNaughton Collins M, Albertsen PC, et al. Comparison of recommendations by urologists and radiation oncologists for treatment of clinically localized prostate cancer. JAMA 2000;283(24):3217–22.
9. Elstein AS. Heuristics and biases: selected errors in clinical reasoning. Acad Med 1999;74(7):791–4.
10. Hogarth RM, Karelaia N. Heuristic and linear models of judgment: matching rules and environments. Psychol Rev 2007;114(3):733–58.
11. Fu AZ, Cantor SB, Kattan MW. Use of nomograms for personalized decision-analytic recommendations. Med Decis Making 2010;30(2):267–74.
12. Saritas I. Prediction of breast cancer using artificial neural networks. J Med Syst 2011 Aug 12. [Epub ahead of print].
13. Biglarian A, Hajizadeh E, Kazemnejad A, et al. Determining of prognostic factors in gastric cancer patients using artificial neural networks. Asian Pac J Cancer Prev 2010;11(2):533–6.
14. Ronco AL, Fernandez R. Improving ultrasonographic diagnosis of prostate cancer with neural networks. Ultrasound Med Biol 1999;25(5):729–33.
15. Kattan MW. Comparison of Cox regression with other methods for determining prediction models and nomograms. J Urol 2003;170:S6–9.
16. Gallina A, Chun FK, Briganti A, et al. Development and split-sample validation of a nomogram predicting the probability of seminal vesicle invasion at radical prostatectomy. Eur Urol 2007;52:98–105.
17. Ross PL, Gerigk C, Gonen M, et al. Comparisons of nomograms and urologists' predictions in prostate cancer. Semin Urol Oncol 2002;20(2):82–8.
18. Morita T, Tsunoda J, Inoue S, et al. Improved accuracy of physicians' survival prediction for terminally ill cancer patients using the palliative prognostic index. Palliat Med 2001;15(5):419–24.
19. Specht MC, Kattan MW, Gonen M, et al. Predicting nonsentinel node status after positive sentinel lymph biopsy for breast cancer: clinicians versus nomogram. Ann Surg Oncol 2005;12(8):654–9.

20. Pound CR, Partin AW, Epstein JI, et al. Prostate-specific antigen after anatomic radical retropubic prostatectomy. Patterns of recurrence and cancer control. Urol Clin North Am 1997;24(2):395–406.
21. Partin AW, Mangold LA, Lamm DM, et al. Contemporary update of prostate cancer staging nomograms (Partin tables) for the new millennium. Urology 2001;58:843.
22. Partin AW, Yoo J, Carter HB, et al. The use of prostate specific antigen, clinical stage and Gleason score to predict pathological stage in men with localized prostate cancer. J Urol 1993;150:110.
23. Partin AW, Kattan MW, Subong EN, et al. Combination of prostate-specific antigen, clinical stage, and Gleason score to predict pathological stage of localized prostate cancer. A multi-institutional update. JAMA 1997;277:1445.
24. Hegedus L. Clinical practice. The thyroid nodule. N Engl J Med 2004;351: 1764–71.
25. Nixon IJ, Ganly I, Hann LE, et al. Nomogram for predicting malignancy in thyroid nodules using clinical, biochemical, ultrasonographic, and cytologic features. Surgery 2010;148(6):1120–7.
26. Okihara K, Nakanishi H, Nakamura T, et al. Clinical characteristics of prostate cancer in Japanese men in the eras before and after serum prostate-specific antigen testing. Int J Urol 2005;12(7):662–7.
27. Ung JO, Richie JP, Chen MH, et al. Evolution of the presentation and pathologic and biochemical outcomes after radical prostatectomy for patients with clinically localized prostate cancer diagnosed during the PSA era. Urology 2002;60(3): 458–63.
28. Kattan MW, Eastham JA, Stapleton AM, et al. A preoperative nomogram for disease recurrence following radical prostatectomy for prostate cancer. J Natl Cancer Inst 1998;90(10):766–71.
29. Kattan MW, Wheeler TM, Scardino PT. Postoperative nomogram for disease recurrence after radical prostatectomy for prostate cancer. J Clin Oncol 1999; 17(5):1499–507.
30. Stephenson AJ, Scardino PT, Eastham JA, et al. Preoperative nomogram predicting the 10-year probability of prostate cancer recurrence after radical prostatectomy. J Natl Cancer Inst 2006;98(10):715–7.
31. Isbarn H, Karakiewicz PI, Walz J, et al. External validation of a preoperative nomogram for prediction of the risk of recurrence after radical prostatectomy. Int J Radiat Oncol Biol Phys 2010;77(3):788–92.
32. Swanson GP, Yu C, Kattan MW, et al. Validation of postoperative nomograms in prostate cancer patients with long-term follow-up. Urology 2011;78(1):105–9.
33. Gill S, Loprinzi CL, Sargent DJ, et al. Pooled analysis of fluorouracil-based adjuvant therapy for stage II and III colon cancer: who benefits and by how much? J Clin Oncol 2004;22(10):1797–806.
34. Cooperberg MR, Carroll PR, Klotz L. Active surveillance for prostate cancer: progress and promise. J Clin Oncol 2011;29(27):3669–76.
35. Kattan MW. Comparative effectiveness: a table of expected benefits and harms. Med Decis Making 2009;29(6):NP3–5.

Randomized Controlled Trials in Surgical Oncology: Where Do We Stand?

Kellie L. Mathis, MD*, Heidi Nelson, MD

KEYWORDS

- Randomized controlled trial • Surgery • Oncology • Rectal cancer

KEY POINTS

- Clinical trials take a long time to mature and they often slow practice innovation, can be contradictory, and are resource intense, requiring a long time and heavy financial commitment.
- Breast cancer trials have guided surgeons to allow for less radical surgery, the separation of the management of the primary tumor from that of the regional disease in the axilla, and they have expanded the role of adjuvant therapies.
- Many surgical advances in rectal cancer occurred before the acceptance and availability of clinical trials.

INTRODUCTION

Providing a summary on clinic trials in surgical oncology is challenging for several reasons. First, the reader is likely to be familiar with the content of concluded trials. Readers have probably changed their practices based on the trials discussed later. Second, a list of currently open trials would provide an uninteresting review and would likely be outdated by the time of printing. The clinical trial has become the accepted gold standard and the basis for numerous evidence-based guidelines that shape clinical practice, so how can an article add value when the readers already have a rich experience with clinical trials in surgical oncology and they can electronically access lists of relevant trials? We say that, to achieve the goal of adding value, we must explore the past to predict the future.

What impact have clinical trials made as individual contributions to knowledge and as a collective influence on how change in surgery is approached? Most who have worked in health care for 10 to 20 years have seen incremental but pervasive changes in how clinicians practice, from emphasis on the individual practitioner's experience and perspective to the more global and specific approach fueled by Cochrane Reviews, meta-analyses, and clinical trials. Practice guidelines and accreditation

Department of Surgery, Division of Colon and Rectal Surgery, Mayo Clinic, 200 First Street SW, Rochester, MN 55905, USA
* Corresponding author.
E-mail address: mathis.kellie@mayo.edu

Surg Oncol Clin N Am 21 (2012) 449–466
doi:10.1016/j.soc.2012.03.002
1055-3207/12/$ – see front matter © 2012 Elsevier Inc. All rights reserved.

standards, as with most advances in medicine, can be seen as a mixed blessing. They bring undesirable conformity, closing a period in which the individual practitioner had more freedom to work individually with patients, but guidelines based on evidence offer the potential for reducing liabilities and improving the safety and quality of practices (if guidelines are practiced uniformly). We say that the value added in reviewing this topic is the opportunity to examine lessons learned from the experiences with clinical trials that have fueled practice-changing evidence. How did this transformation in practice happen, what role did clinical trials play in the past, and what role are they likely to play in the future? What were the intended and unintended consequences of clinical trials? In addition, this article also addresses the vulnerabilities of practicing based on clinical trial evidence and how these vulnerabilities might be addressed in the future.

CLINICAL TRIALS: ARE THEY RELEVANT IN SURGERY?

The first perception that should be dispelled is that clinical trials do not play a significant role in surgery and that surgeons have not played a significant role in clinical trials. This perception may be true if one simply quantitates the percentage of surgical practice that is driven by clinical trials results. A study by Howes and colleagues[1] in the United Kingdom in 1997 suggested that, in medicine, clinical trial evidence was integrated into 50% of clinical practice, whereas in surgery only 24% of the practice was based on evidence. From a quantitative standpoint, clinical trial evidence in surgery is not as pervasive as for medicine. There is likely always to be some discrepancy between medicine and surgery with respect to the extent of evidence, because medications all require the approval of the US Food and Drug Administrations (FDA), so substantial data must be gathered for each new drug and for each disease-specific indication. No such scrutiny and oversight is required for surgery. All new devices must undergo FDA approval for their stated objective (eg, tissue destruction, stapling, laparoscopic visualization). However, once a device is approved based on evidence that it can perform such functions, it can move swiftly from one site or discipline to another (eg, from an application in bowel to an application in lung). The evidence that is required by law for surgical advances is minimal, and there are few national drivers for surgical research.

Further complicating the situation is that, to examine surgery requires measurement and monitoring of the technical aspects of surgical procedures. This highly expensive endeavor is beyond what government agencies can afford or achieve. Despite this, there is a rich legacy of surgeon-driven science. It was arguably surgeons in the surgical group National Surgical Adjuvant Breast and Bowel Project (NSABP) who greatly changed the practice of breast cancer care. The first part of this article details the lessons learned from breast cancer trials with a summation of both progress made and limitations experienced.

BREAST CANCER TRIALS: A RADICAL IMPACT ON PRACTICE

This first story follows a series of breast cancer trials that challenged the radical mastectomy and transformed the practice of breast cancer care. The story starts with Halsted,[2] who described the radical mastectomy in the 1890s. This technique persisted into the 1970s, in large part because surgery was the only therapy available. Consequently, resection of the breast and adjacent axillary tissues and/or adherent structures such as the chest wall made sense for patients with breast cancer given the limited options and the lethality of the disease. Any residual disease, visible or microscopic, was known to result in certain recurrence and likely death. As the story evolved over several decades, it was in the context of the safety and rigor of clinical trials, that this radical approach could be challenged in favor of less extensive surgery and with the adoption of other local-regional and systemic therapies.

To the best of our ability to ascertain, the first studies to challenge the standard but radical nature of the Halsted mastectomy were initiated in London in the 1960s. These early studies may have introduced the concept of breast conservation, but they showed increased mortality for breast-conserving therapy.[3] These initial suboptimal results rendered it difficult to proceed with additional trials on the same subject. Despite this obstacle, a Milan trial, designed to compare outcomes from the Halsted radical mastectomy with quadrantectomy, was approved and began to accrue patients in 1969. Results were published in 1981 and established the safety of breast-conserving therapy.[4–6]

Several lessons were learned in this early experience. First, clinical trials take a long time to mature and so they slow the process of practice innovation, particularly when the stakes and the degree of uncertainty are high. Second, trials can be contradictory, a problem that continues to be true even today. For those 2 reasons, it is common for most practice-changing trials to be repeated at least once. Just like an experiment in a laboratory, repetition is important for confirming results and creating confidence in the finding. When trial results are not concordant, it is usually because of imperfect understanding of the clinical trials or difference in design. A series of carefully designed trials sequentially migrated the care of the patient with breast cancer from radical mastectomy to the era of breast-conserving therapy and the introduction of radiation and chemotherapy (described later in the article).

In the United States, Fisher and colleagues[7] from 1971 to 1974 randomized 1079 women with clinically node-negative breast cancer to radical mastectomy, total mastectomy, and total mastectomy with nodal radiation therapy. They found no difference in overall survival, disease-free survival, recurrence-free survival, or distant metastasis. They also randomized 586 node-positive patients to radical mastectomy versus total mastectomy with radiation therapy and found no difference in survival. These results remained true after 25 years of follow-up,[8] as did the results of 20-year follow-up in the Veronisi Italian study.[9,10] This finding led to the conclusion that there was no survival benefit to radical mastectomy, and the radical standard was abandoned in favor of a new, less invasive procedure. The safety net of testing less invasive procedures in breast cancer was the emerging role of radiation therapy. From this point forward, radiation played a more prominent role in the care of the patient with breast cancer.

The next clinical question postulated was whether total mastectomy could be replaced with a less invasive alternative, lumpectomy. Fisher and colleagues[11–14] randomized patients with operable cancers that were less than 4 cm in size to lumpectomy plus axillary dissection, lumpectomy plus axillary dissection and radiation therapy, and radical mastectomy. They found a lower local recurrence in the group of patients with lumpectomy plus radiation therapy compared with lumpectomy alone (14 vs 39%). There was no difference in overall survival, disease-free survival, and distant metastasis across all groups.[11–14]

These 3 studies (Milan study, NSABP B-04, and B-06)[5,12,15] led to the acceptance of breast-conserving therapy plus radiation therapy as a method of treatment. In addition, total mastectomy or lumpectomy plus radiation therapy were preferred to radical mastectomy.

After accepting breast-conserving therapy as a viable option for management of the primary tumor, multiple international studies showed that radiation therapy in addition to the lumpectomy or quadrantectomy resulted in improved local control. It was again shown that radiation therapy did not offer any survival advantage compared with surgery alone.[16–20] This finding confirms that radiation, like surgery, is a local-regional therapy. There has never been evidence that radiation therapy could replace surgery altogether, even in cases of complete clinical response after neoadjuvant chemoradiation therapy.

Another line of investigation focused on whether combining one local-regional therapy and a systemic therapy (hormonal therapy with tamoxifen) could be superior to 2 local-regional therapies (surgery and radiation therapy). The NSABP B-21 trial studied whether tamoxifen could be as effective as radiation therapy at controlling ipsilateral disease after lumpectomy in tumors less than 1cm in size. This trial randomized 1009 women after lumpectomy and axillary lymph node dissection (ALND) to tamoxifen alone, radiation therapy plus tamoxifen, or radiation therapy plus placebo. The addition of radiation therapy to lumpectomy was better (local recurrence 9%) than tamoxifen alone (local recurrence 16%) at controlling local ipsilateral disease, and the addition of both tamoxifen and radiation therapy was the best (local recurrence 3%), regardless of the patient's hormone receptor status.[21] This finding led to the conclusion that tamoxifen and radiation therapy should be considered even in tumors of less than 1 cm. A similar study by Fyles and colleagues[22] showed similar results: tamoxifen plus radiation therapy improved local and regional control with no difference in overall or disease-free survival. The Cancer and Leukemia Group B (CALGB) group randomized 636 patients older than 70 years with T1N0 estrogen receptor–positive tumors to lumpectomy with tamoxifen only or lumpectomy with tamoxifen and radiation therapy. Local recurrence with tamoxifen alone was 4% versus 1% in the group that received tamoxifen and radiation therapy (statistically significant). There was no difference in overall survival. The investigators concluded that tamoxifen alone after breast-conserving therapy in women more than 70 years old with small estrogen receptor–positive tumors may be considered for a radiation-sparing treatment.[23] With the effort to reduce the use of radiation therapy, systemic therapy has been introduced as a new standard in patients with early-stage disease.

Given the additive benefits of systemic therapy, the logical next step was to add chemotherapy regimens with demonstrated survival benefits in stage IV patients. The NSABP B-20 trial randomized 2306 women to chemotherapy plus tamoxifen versus tamoxifen alone, and the addition of chemotherapy resulted in improved disease-free survival, overall survival, and local recurrence.[24] Therefore, both hormonal therapy and chemotherapy should be considered. A similar study was done in postmenopausal women. This study also showed a trend toward improved overall and disease-free survival for patients receiving both tamoxifen and chemotherapy.[25]

The surgical approach to the primary tumor had been maximally reduced to achieve the greatest degree of breast conservation. However, little progress had been made toward reducing other morbidity, such as lymphedema from axillary dissection. Once systemic therapy was affecting survival, it became possible to consider reducing the radical nature of the surgical management of lymph nodes. A first step toward decreasing the radical nature of breast cancer staging (sentinel lymph node biopsy [SLNB]) was promoted by Krag and colleagues[26,27] as part of the NSABP B-32 study. They randomized 5611 women with clinically node-negative disease into SLNB followed by immediate ALND versus SLNB alone (ALND only performed if a positive lymph node was found on SLNB). The technical success rate of the SLNB was 97%, with a mean number of 2.1 lymph nodes removed. The SLN-positive rate was also 26% in both groups. When the SLN was negative, the ALND was also negative in 96% for an overall accuracy of 95%. The overall false-negative rate was 10%. In the 26% of SLN-positive patients who went on to ALND, 61% had no further positive disease.[26,27] The conclusion of the study was that the SLN accuracy rate is high. The

Sentinella Italian study[28] had a similar design. The local recurrence rate in the ALND group was 1% versus 5% in the SLNB group (axillary recurrence in 0 vs 1 patient). The SLNB group had less lymphedema, mobility restrictions, and numbness. Additional studies were done confirming less lymphedema and numbness in the SLNB group.[29,30] The Milan study randomized more than 1000 patients to SLNB alone versus SLNB with immediate ALND and found axillary failures in 0.0004% of the SLNB group versus 0% in the ALND group, with no difference in overall survival or distant metastasis.[31]

Following these studies, SLNB replaced ALND as the technique of choice to stage the disease. To further expand the role of reducing the extent of surgery, patients who were found to have 1 or 2 positive axillary nodes on the SLNB were randomized to completion ALND or no further surgery in the American College of Surgeons Oncology Group (ACOSOG) Z0011 trial. The investigators found no difference in overall or disease-free survival between the groups, suggesting that ALND may be spared in some women with limited nodal disease.[32]

As experience with breast cancer trials grew, there came a realization that breast cancer is a systemic disease and that the risk of systemic failure was more threatening than the risk of local failure. This mentality likely fueled the transition from postoperative adjuvant chemotherapy to neoadjuvant trials. The NSABP B-18 trial randomized 1523 women with T1-T3, N0-N1 tumors to preoperative chemotherapy (doxorubicin and cyclophosphamide [AC]) in patients with operable disease versus postoperative chemotherapy (AC). There was a high clinical response rate in the neoadjuvant group and 9% of patients had a pathologic complete response. There was also nodal downstaging as well as a higher rate of breast-conserving therapy in this group. There was no difference in survival between the preoperative and postoperative chemotherapy groups, but an improvement in survival was seen in the group with a pathologic complete response.[33] The 16-year update to this study concluded that neoadjuvant chemotherapy is comparable with adjuvant AC and may allow breast-conserving therapy for patients who would otherwise require mastectomy.[34] Additional trials examined the role of neoadjuvant aromatase inhibitor therapy in postmenopausal women to increase the incidence of breast-conserving therapy. In the ACOSOG Z1031 trial, 51% of those deemed candidates for mastectomy only at presentation were able to undergo breast-conserving therapy after neoadjuvant therapy.[35] Neoadjuvant also allows a window to judge response to chemotherapy and/or hormonal therapy before the tumor is removed, which may have implications for postoperative adjuvant therapy.

Trials are also being used to validate multigene assays for risk assessment. The Oncotype DX is a diagnostic panel of 21 genes. It has been shown to accurately predict the likelihood of distant recurrence in women with node-negative, estrogen receptor–positive tumors in a subgroup of 668 patients from the NSABP B-14 trial.[36]

A summary of biologic and therapeutic lessons learned from breast cancer trials described the progression from the Halsted radical mastectomy to breast-conserving therapy in most women diagnosed in the modern era. The randomized controlled trials (RCTs) have allowed the separation of management of the primary tumor in the breast from the management of the regional disease in the axilla, preparing for SLNB as a means of staging, which led to decreased morbidity and less radical surgery. In addition, the RCTs expanded the role of adjuvant therapies for the treatment of breast cancer. Radiation therapy is now considered essential in most patients, but it is becoming apparent that it may be safely avoided in the future in select patients (women more than 70 years old with small tumors).[23] The role of neoadjuvant and adjuvant chemotherapies has expanded greatly in the last few decades. In the recent past, RCTs in breast cancer also introduced the concepts of gene sequencing and biomarkers that will help to individualize treatments for each patient. In addition, trials require a long time and large financial commitment from the participating surgeon, and all trials with significant positive or negative findings are generally repeated to confirm the results, often in a different geographic region.

BREAST CANCER: THE LIMITATIONS OF CLINICAL TRIALS

As mentioned earlier, trials inform a minority of clinical surgical practices (roughly 25%). Trials are expensive and time consuming. To properly address a clinical question through a clinical trial costs tens of millions of dollars. The larger the study and the more complicated the trial, the more costly it will be. At a minimum, cancer trials cost on the order of $6000 per patient for enrollment. When diagnostic or therapeutic components that are not standard of care are added, then these costs must be covered by research funding. Sources of funding from government agencies are limited because of competition across many health care sectors. Sources of funding for surgical trials from industry are not as abundant as those in medical fields. Pharmaceutical companies support drug development and clinical testing for FDA filing on a routine basis. Surgeons often have fewer options and must seek creative solutions, although these are available.

Two other limitations deserve to be mentioned. The first is a long period of time from trial results to practice to semination, and the second is the severe discrepancy between the number of patients tested in trials and the number treated in practice. Limitations may be interrelated and so are discussed together.

The lag time from trial reporting to full practice implementation is 17 years. Reasons for this extreme lag time are not completely elucidated. Further, it is not known whether this lag time is beneficial or detrimental, or even whether it is uniform across different studies and practices. It is assumed that the lag time is detrimental, which may be true for therapies that are life saving, low risk, and easy to administer. It is logical that a delay in implementation would be detrimental under these conditions. However, this might not be a reliable assumption where there is a marginal gain from a newly introduced therapy. A marginal gain could be lost if there are only moderate benefits to be gained, and there is potential for real risks because of a lack of experience with the new therapy. For example, after the introduction of laparoscopic cholecystectomy, the rates of common bile duct injuries and lawsuits increased significantly because of the rapid adoption of the procedure. The laparoscopic cholecystectomy was adopted into practice before any formal testing and postgraduate training were available. A marginal benefit could be readily lost if a new practice is widely adopted by practitioners in the absence of standard safety measures inherent in clinical trials.

Clinical trials have several safety measures to protect the patient and practitioners from excessive and unnecessary risk. This safety net starts with narrow eligibility criteria so that sick, frail, at-risk patients are not included in trials. These eligibility criteria are often neglected when the results are reported and practices start to implement new recommendations. Further safety measures and procedures for monitoring and managing toxicities are well defined in trials and help guide clinicians participating in trials. Data safety monitoring boards supervise the trial to be certain the collective experience is following a safe procedure. Could the newness of the procedure or medication, coupled with the absence of these safety mechanisms, be the reason for slow adoption of such therapies and practice? Any drug or procedure that is not familiar to the practitioner should be approached with caution. Future efforts to specifically address critical transitions from trials to practice could benefit all parties.

Further deterrence for early adoption could relate to major discrepancies between the 3% of patients who participate in trials and the remaining 97% who might or might not benefit from the therapy recommended by the trial results. Trial reporting is often considered the final step in the research process and is left to the pharmaceutical company or the principal investigator to disseminate the news and help with implementation of the new standard. The hand-off to practitioners is poor at best. Nuances in the trial design, eligibility, and findings are often difficult to sort through without the explicit aid of the study team. There is no official support for the study team or for the structured dissemination of the findings into practice after the trial is reported. Little is known about the potential for unintended consequences from the introduction of new standards into practice. Before rushing to reduce the 17-year dissemination lag, tools are needed to measure and monitor this process.

RECTAL CANCER TRIALS

With abundant lessons learned in breast cancer, we considered whether the same lessons could apply to another field of investigation. We chose to review rectal cancer because of the similarities in who funds these cancer trials (eg, National Cancer Institute and pharmaceutical companies) and how they are typically conducted. They are dissimilar based on the many anatomic, physiologic, and biologic differences between the 2 diseases. The story of rectal cancer trials starts later than breast cancer trials and after major changes in surgical techniques (ie, sphincter preservation) had evolved.

Before the nineteenth century, rectal cancer was considered incurable. Attempts to resect rectal tumors resulted in perioperative death or certain early recurrence. With advances in anesthesia and asepsis in the late 1800s, surgery rapidly moved to become a potentially curative therapy for rectal cancer. Radical abdominal perineal resections (APR) for rectal cancer were described by Miles[37] in 1908; APR remains one of the standard, curative approaches to rectal cancer care. The challenge for the APR as an oncologic therapy is the radical transformation it imposes on patients. Sphincter-saving operations were then proposed for tumors of the upper rectum in the 1940s by Claude Dixon[38] at the Mayo Clinic after he showed no difference in survival at 5 years between patients with tumors 16 to 20 cm from the dentate line and tumors 6 to 10 cm from the dentate. This work was followed by technical advancements and the development of surgical staplers as well as evidence of cure rates, leading to the expansion of sphincter-sparing surgery to include middle and lower rectal tumors. These radical changes from APR for all patients to sphincter-sparing surgery for most occurred outside clinical trials.

These sphincter-sparing procedures were adopted widely over time and studied only retrospectively. As new procedures became technically possible (eg, staplers allowed the possibility of sphincter-sparing low anterior resection), questions arose, such as what constituted adequate margins. Reports from observational studies initially supported a 5-cm distal bowel margin, but subsequent studies (nonrandomized) suggested that the traditional 5-cm requirement was not necessary and mucosal margins of between 1 and 2 cm were acceptable.[39] Each time incremental advances in surgical technique were achieved, oncologic outcomes were disputed, and new practices gradually emerged. Advances were supported by the publishing of institutional series. By the 1970s, the field was evolving to include not only surgery but to also include options to participate in experimental protocols that involved the administration of adjuvant radiation therapy.

Because of the poor survival rates in patients with local-regional disease who were treated with surgery alone, investigators questioned whether the addition of radiation therapy could improve the results. Sentinel radiation trials found that postoperative external beam radiation decreased local recurrence rates compared with surgery alone. The NSABP R-01 trial randomized 555 patients with Dukes B and C tumors from 1977 to 1986 into 3 arms following surgery: observation, chemotherapy only (5-fluorouracil, semustine, and vincristine), or radiation therapy only (46–47 Gy). There was an improvement in the local recurrence rate in the radiation therapy arm (25% vs 16%, $P = .06$) but no difference in overall or disease-free survival. The chemotherapy arm showed an improvement in overall and disease-free survival.[40] In the Medical Research Council Rectal Cancer Working Party study, 469 British and Irish patients were randomized to surgery alone or surgery followed by radiation therapy (42 Gy) from 1984 to 1989. There was no difference in overall survival ($P = .17$) or disease-free survival ($P = .18$), but there was a benefit with regard to local recurrence (34% vs 21%, hazard ratio 0.54, $P = .001$). Side effects were well-tolerated and late events were rare.[41] Many similar trials were performed, including NSABP R-02,[42] Denmark study,[43] and the Gastrointestinal Tumor Study Group,[44] and all confirmed that postoperative adjuvant radiation contributes to local-regional control.[45]

A meta-analysis of 22 randomized trials (n = 8507 patients) comparing any radiation for rectal cancer (before or after surgery) with surgery alone and found no difference in overall survival (62% vs 63%, $P = .06$) but a statistically significant reduction in local recurrence rates with radiation therapy.[46]

The parallel clinical question was whether the addition of chemotherapy to radiation would add survival benefit. Krook and colleagues[47] randomized 204 patients from 1980 to 1986 to postoperative radiation therapy (50.4 Gy) versus postoperative chemoradiation therapy (9 weeks of 5-fluorouracil and methyl-CCNU followed by 50.4-Gy radiation therapy with concurrent 5-fluorouracil, followed by an additional 9 weeks of 5-fluorouracil and CCNU). The 5-year overall recurrence in the radiation therapy alone group was 63% versus 41% in the chemoradiation therapy group. Local recurrence (25% vs 13%) and distant metastasis rates (46% vs 29%) were also improved with the addition of chemotherapy, as was overall survival. This study confirmed that chemotherapy combined with radiation therapy was superior to radiation therapy alone. This finding led to a new standard of care that persists today: radiation therapy should be given concurrently with chemotherapy. The National Institutes of Health consensus conference in 1990 recommended postoperative chemoradiation therapy as the standard of care for patients with T3 and T4 tumors as well as for those with nodal disease. Patients with stage I and II disease were observed.[48]

If postoperative chemoradiation was improving survival, investigators next asked whether neoadjuvant radiation could further improve outcomes. The next set of clinical trials was varied in design because some compared neoadjuvant radiation with surgery alone and others compared neoadjuvant therapy with postoperative radiation therapy. Some trials examined short-course radiation and others used standard-course radiation therapy. The European Organization for Research and Treatment of Cancer randomized 466 patients to surgery alone versus preoperative radiation therapy. They found no survival difference but improved local recurrence rates (30% vs 15%).[49] The Stockholm I trial randomized 849 patients to preoperative short-course radiation therapy versus surgery alone from 1980 to 1987. The local recurrence rate and time to failure was better in the neoadjuvant group but, again, no benefit in overall survival was established.[50] An additional finding was a higher postoperative mortality in the group that received preoperative radiation therapy (8% vs 2%).

The Stockholm II trial randomized 557 patients to short-course radiation therapy plus surgery versus surgery alone. In this study, the radiation therapy group benefited in local recurrence, distant metastasis, and overall survival.[51] The Swedish Rectal Cancer Trial also randomized 1168 patients to preoperative short-course radiation therapy versus surgery alone. At the 13-year follow-up, there was an improved overall survival (38% vs 30%) as well as local recurrence rate (9% vs 26%).[52] Follow-up results from this trial showed that morbidity was higher in the neoadjuvant radiation group, specifically the rate of small bowel obstruction.[53] The United Kingdom study, from 1998 to 2005, randomized 1350 patients to preoperative short-course radiation therapy versus postoperative chemoradiation therapy (5-fluorouracil and leucovorin). They found an improved local recurrence rate in the preoperative radiation therapy group (4 vs 11%). The disease-free survival was also higher in the group receiving neoadjuvant radiation therapy (77 vs 71%); no difference was seen in overall survival.[54]

A German trial randomized 823 patients from 1995 to 2002 to preoperative versus postoperative long-course radiation therapy plus 5-fluorouracil. They found no difference in overall or disease-free survival but a local recurrence rate (6% vs 13%) that benefited from neoadjuvant therapy. There was less acute and late toxicity in the preoperative group (but fewer patients in the postoperative group received complete radiation therapy; 54% vs 92%).[55] Many other studies[56,57] showed similar results with decreased local recurrence rates in groups who received preoperative radiation therapy. Camma and colleagues[58] performed a meta-analysis of all randomized trials that compared preoperative radiation therapy plus surgery and surgery alone; neoadjuvant radiation therapy resulted in improved 5-year overall survival and cancer-specific survival as well as lowered local recurrence rates, but the magnitude of the benefit was small. The summative results of these trials led to the conclusion that neoadjuvant radiation therapy is superior to surgery alone and superior to postoperative radiation therapy.

A unique byproduct from these trials was the recognition that local recurrence rates were variable among the studies. This finding led investigators to focus more on the role of surgical technique, specifically the management of the perirectal lymphatic packet (ie, mesorectum). The Dutch trial was the first to require surgeons to perform standardized surgery (total mesorectal excision [TME]) in all trial patients. Patients were randomized to preoperative short-course radiation therapy plus TME versus TME alone. The local recurrence rate at 2 years was 2.4% versus 8.2%, favoring radiation therapy, but no difference was seen in overall survival.[59] The long-term follow-up at 5 years showed the same results with local recurrence rates: 11% versus 6% favoring radiation therapy and no difference in overall survival.[60] The 10-year follow-up results were similar.[61]

As for breast cancer trials, efforts transitioned from local-regional treatments to more systemic treatment. The next clinical question was therefore whether the addition of chemotherapy to the neoadjuvant radiation therapy regimen would add benefit. Bosset and colleagues[62] randomized 1011 patients to preoperative radiation therapy alone, preoperative radiation plus 5-fluorouracil, preoperative radiation therapy plus postoperative 5-fluorouracil, or preoperative radiation plus postoperative 5-fluorouracil. There was a benefit to local control with 5-fluorouracil chemotherapy given at any time point compared with radiation therapy alone. No survival benefit was seen. The Polish study randomized 312 patients to short-course neoadjuvant radiation therapy only versus long-course neoadjuvant radiation therapy plus 5-fluorouracil. There was no difference in disease-free or overall survival, sphincter preservation, or complications. There were more early toxicities in the chemoradiation therapy group.[63]

A French study group randomized 733 patients to preoperative radiation therapy alone versus preoperative radiation therapy with 5-fluorouracil. No difference was seen in overall survival or sphincter preservation, but there was an improvement in the local recurrence rate in the chemoradiation therapy group (8% vs 16%). However, this improvement was balanced by higher toxicity in this group.[64]

A systematic review of 5 RCTs comparing preoperative chemoradiation therapy versus preoperative radiation therapy alone confirmed higher pathologic complete response rates in the chemoradiation therapy group, but this was balanced by higher toxicity.[65]

Following these trials, the algorithm for treating rectal cancer changed further to offer neoadjuvant chemoradiation therapy to patients with bulky T3 tumors, all T4 tumors, and all with suspected nodal disease. Postoperative radiation therapy is reserved for patients who have one of these findings unexpectedly at the time of surgery.

Many RCTs have attempted to determine the value of adjuvant 5-fluorouracil–based chemotherapy following surgery for rectal cancer, but there is unclear benefit in the current available literature (4 total randomized trials). The consensus from the systematic review combining these 4 trials is that additional trials are needed to answer this question.[66]

Although many of the surgical advances in rectal cancer care occurred before the acceptance and availability of clinical trial methodology, the same was not true for the introduction of laparoscopic techniques. When the minimally invasive surgical approach to abdominal disorders became a technical reality, it radically changed the management of the gallbladder. As it was considered for the colon application, it was resisted in oncologic cases. The frequent reporting of port-site recurrences slowed the advancement of laparoscopic surgery for colon cancer until international trials showed the same oncologic outcomes for laparoscopic as for open surgery. Once laparoscopic colectomy for cancer was proved safe and effective, it prompted similar studies in rectal cancer. Many centers considered the possibility of laparoscopic surgery following the same oncologic principles accepted in open rectal cancer surgery.[67] The Conventional Versus Laparoscopic-Assisted Surgery in Patients with Colorectal Cancer (CLASICC) trial included patients with benign and malignant rectal disease (48% had rectal cancers). Laparoscopy shortened the length of hospital stay but resulted in a higher rate of positive circumferential resection margins (12% vs 6%) and worse sexual function in male patients. There were no significant differences in local recurrence, 3-year disease-free survival, and overall survival.[68–70]

Lujan and colleagues[71] conducted a single-institution study and reported results from their randomized trial that compared open and laparoscopic surgery for rectal cancer in 204 patients. They found no difference in local recurrence, disease-free survival, or overall survival and no difference in involvement of the circumferential resection margins. Additional trials are ongoing to further explore the role of laparoscopy in rectal cancer surgery. ACOSOG Z6051 is a noninferiority trial with endpoints that include number of patients with circumferential resection margins less than 1 mm, distal margin greater than 2 cm, and completeness of TME. Similar trials are in progress in other countries (UK CLASICC, COLOR II, Japan Clinical Oncology Group [JCOG] 0404). Results of these trials are not yet available, and open rectal cancer surgery remains the standard.

Attempts to decrease the radical nature of surgery in patients with early rectal cancer have included local excision techniques (transanal excision and transanal endoscopic microsurgery [TEM]). Many series have been reported but few trials have tested the safety and oncologic benefit of local excision. The study by Lezoche and colleagues[72] randomized 70 patients with T2N0 rectal tumors to TEM versus laparoscopic TME (both groups received neoadjuvant radiation therapy and 5-fluorouracil). With a median follow-up of 84 months, there were no differences in local recurrence rates, rates of distant metastases, or survival outcomes. This study was underpowered to detect small differences in these outcomes. Winde and colleagues[73] randomized 50 patients to anterior resection versus transanal endoscopic microsurgery; there were similar local recurrence and survival rates and decreased morbidity in the TEM group.

However, long-term prospective studies from Memorial Sloan Kettering[74] and the University of Minnesota[75] have shown worse outcomes for the local excision groups when they were followed over time. Additional data from the National Cancer Database suggest that, although the use of local excision techniques has increased greatly, the risk of local recurrence at 5 years was 12.5% for T1 tumors and 22.1% for T2 tumors.[76] An ongoing multi-institutional study, ACOSOG Z6041, follows patients with T2N0 low rectal tumors who were given radiation therapy and capecitabine and oxaliplatin before surgery followed by local excision. If the pathology confirms T0 to T2 disease, the patient is observed and, if T3 or positive margins remain, the patient undergoes further treatment. It remains to be determined whether local excision should be considered for rectal cancers, but the treatment algorithm in the 2010s may include local excision in select patients with T1N0 disease.

RECTAL CANCER TRIALS: SUMMARY

A summary of lessons learned from the rectal cancer trials described includes the progression from surgery alone for all rectal tumors with resultant high recurrence rates to the current management of adjuvant chemotherapy and radiation therapy, preferably done in a neoadjuvant sequence. Attempts to minimize the radical nature of surgery are ongoing with the possible acceptance of laparoscopy pending the results of ongoing trials as well as local excision techniques for very early and favorable histology tumors. In contrast with breast cancer management, the separation of the treatment of the primary disease from treatment/staging of the regional lymph nodes has yet to accomplished in rectal cancer. The axilla and pelvis present different challenges for nodal sampling. Trials are usually repeated across multiple institutions and countries to confirm the results.

ADDITIONAL LESSONS LEARNED FROM SURGICAL CLINICAL TRIALS

Another important topic is how new techniques that are shown through trials to be equivalent or superior to the prior gold standard are widely introduced and implemented into surgical practices. The historical approach of see 1, do 1, teach 1 is no longer the standard. The ideal educational model designed to educate a postgraduate on a new technique would include structured teaching, verification of necessary knowledge and technical skills using validated and reliable tools, the availability of postcourse preceptoring or proctoring, and diligent monitoring of outcomes.[77] This ideal is difficult to achieve because of the time and financial resources that are required.

Two examples of wide implementation of new surgical procedures are the SLNB in breast cancer and TME in rectal cancer. After clinical trials proved the safety and efficacy of the SLNB,[78] a consensus statement from the American Society of Breast Surgeons (ASBS) recommended that surgeons perform a minimum of 30 cases of SLNB combined with ALND and achieve a false-negative rate of 5% or less before using SLNB alone for axillary staging.[79] A study by McMasters and colleagues[80] suggested that 20 SLNBs were required to reach the peak of the learning curve before abandoning axillary dissection. However, the oversight and ultimate decision about who was qualified to perform SLNB came only from individual hospital credentialing boards and was not regulated at the national level.

In rectal cancer surgery, the Dutch experience of training TME confirmed that focused education can improve outcomes. Educational programs included workshops and instructional videos. In some regions, trained instructor surgeons were on site and the first few TME procedures performed in each hospital were supervised. In addition, the quality of the pathologic assessment was monitored by supervising pathologists. The Dutch trial, which compared preoperative radiation therapy and surgery versus surgery alone, required TME in both arms. The local recurrence rates of 2.4% and 8% in the 2 arms[60] compared favorably with the higher recurrence rates reported in studies done before the introduction of TME.

Before surgeons were allowed to participate in the NSABP B-32 trial (comparing SLNB with ALND) they had to complete a prerandomization training phase (ie, credentialing). Training consisted of written materials, direct instruction in the operating room, and immediate feedback. With this intense program, most surgeons required only 5 training cases before they were credentialed to begin randomizing patients.[81] Many of the completed and ongoing surgical clinical trials by the ACOSOG required pretrial credentialing of all surgeons to participate (specifically, ACOSOG Z0010, Z0020, Z0030, Z0360, Z6041, Z4032, Z1072, Z4033, and Z6051).

FUTURE DIRECTIONS ENCOMPASSING LESSONS LEARNED FROM SURGICAL TRIALS

First, great progress is being made in the understanding of the biology of cancer. As an understanding of the biology of each tumor is reached, the treatment of each patient can be individualized. Ongoing studies in breast cancer are looking for particular gene signatures that can predict the likelihood of complete response to neoadjuvant therapies as well as early and late recurrences. Knowing which patients are at risk allows adjuvant therapies to be tailored. New trial designs, like the adaptive ISPY-2 randomized trial that is enrolling patients with locally advanced breast cancer, use individual patient biomarker profiles to tailor neoadjuvant therapies in addition to the standard chemotherapies. As the trial is ongoing, information about how patients with specific biomarkers respond to each novel drug will be used to inform which drugs will be assigned to future patients. Learning occurs quickly as the trial proceeds and the design of the study is adjusted in real time to account for the findings.[82]

The second area that needs to be improved on is the way the gap is bridged from trial results to implementation of new techniques in clinical practice. The first step, pretrial credentialing with specific protocols and procedural guidelines as well as monitoring of adherence to these guidelines during the trial, seems to be the new standard in randomized surgical trials. However, there is no regulation of how the trial results become incorporated into surgical practices. The American College of Surgeons Commission on Cancer Alliance is working on improving the translation of trial to practice. It intends to organize training workshops for dissemination of new techniques using the resources of the American College of Surgeons Accredited Educational Institutes.[83] These workshops would use the credentialing tools used in trials and offer them as measures to evaluate surgeons' technical ability to perform new procedures. Refresher courses and the opportunity for newly trained surgeons to ask questions of the experts should be available. Accreditation standards could eventually be set using validated technical skills evaluation criteria. It may be possible that such accreditation tools could be adopted by the surgical boards. Registries can then be used to perform ongoing monitoring when new procedures are introduced into practice as a tool to examine long-term patient outcomes.

It is clear from this article and others that randomized trials have flaws. Although clinical trials are considered the gold standard for the quality of data obtained, they are not feasible or ethical for all surgical questions. In these cases, observational studies are required. The chief limitation of randomized trials is that they are resource intense and require a lot of time and money to test 1 or 2 hypotheses. In addition, it is assumed that there are no relevant differences between the patients treated in the tightly controlled trial setting and the patients who will be treated in the clinical setting (ie, the ability to generalize). An additional problem in surgical trials is that standardization of surgical techniques is difficult and often requires the coordination of multiple specialties to accomplish (eg, pathology, radiation oncology, medical oncology). Without this standardization, inaccurate conclusions can be drawn, as discussed in a recent editorial by Dr Ko,[84] who made the point that observational studies should be considered complementary. Observational studies can often be completed in less time and with fewer costs. They may be used to generate hypotheses that can then be tested in the context of a randomized trial or can be used to test the external validity or the ability to generalize results from clinical trials. Furthermore, well-designed observational studies that account for possible confounding from the outset may yield data that are of high enough quality to answer difficult surgical questions without the need for a clinical trial. We propose that it may be an ideal time to rethink criteria for optimizing the choice between an observational study and a randomized trial.

REFERENCES

1. Howes N, Chagla L, Thorpe M, et al. Surgical practice is evidence based. Br J Surg 1997;84(9):1220–3.
2. Halsted W. The results of operations for cure of cancer of the breast performed at the John Hopkins Hospital from June 1889 to January 1894. Ann Surg 1894;20(5):297–350.
3. Fentiman I. Long-term follow-up of the first breast conservation trial: Guy' wide excision study. Breast 2000;9(1):5–8.
4. Veronesi U, Saccozzi R, Vecchio MD, et al. Comparing radical mastectomy with quadrantectomy, axillary dissection, and radiotherapy in patients with small cancers of the breast. N Engl J Med 1981;305(1):6–11.
5. Veronesi U, Salvadori B, Luini A, et al. Breast conservation is a safe method in patients with small cancer of the breast. Long-term results of three randomised trials on 1,973 patients. Eur J Cancer 1995;31A(10):1574–9.
6. Veronisi U. Conservative treatment of breast cancer: a trial in progress at the Cancer Institute of Milan. World J Surg 1977;1(3):324–6.
7. Fisher B, Redmond C, Fisher ER, et al. Ten-year results of a randomized clinical trial comparing radical mastectomy and total mastectomy with or without radiation. N Engl J Med 1985;312(11):674–81.
8. Fisher B, Jeong JH, Anderson S, et al. Twenty-five-year follow-up of a randomized trial comparing radical mastectomy, total mastectomy, and total mastectomy followed by irradiation. N Engl J Med 2002;347(8):567–75.
9. Veronesi U, Cascinelli N, Mariani L, et al. Twenty-year follow-up of a randomized study comparing breast-conserving surgery with radical mastectomy for early breast cancer. N Engl J Med 2002;347:1227–32.
10. Fisher B, Costantino J, Redmond C, et al. Lumpectomy compared with lumpectomy and radiation therapy for the treatment of intraductal breast cancer. N Engl J Med 1993;328(22):1581–6.

11. Fisher B, Anderson S, Bryant J, et al. Twenty-year follow-up of a randomized trial comparing total mastectomy, lumpectomy, and lumpectomy plus irradiation for the treatment of invasive breast cancer. N Engl J Med 2002;347(16):1233–41.

12. Fisher B, Bauer M, Margolese R, et al. Five-year results of a randomized clinical trial comparing total mastectomy and segmental mastectomy with or without radiation in the treatment of breast cancer. N Engl J Med 1985;312(11):665–73.

13. Fisher B, Redmond C, Poisson R, et al. Eight-year results of a randomized clinical trial comparing total mastectomy and lumpectomy with or without irradiation in the treatment of breast cancer. N Engl J Med 1989;320(13):822–8.

14. Fisher B, Anderson S, Redmond CK, et al. Reanalysis and results after 12 years of follow-up in a randomized clinical trial comparing total mastectomy with lumpectomy with or without irradiation in the treatment of breast cancer. N Engl J Med 1995;333(22):1456–61.

15. Fisher B, Montague E, Redmond C, et al. Comparison of radical mastectomy with alternative treatments for primary breast cancer. A first report of results from a prospective randomized clinical trial. Cancer 1977;39(Suppl 6):2827–39.

16. Liljegren G, Holmberg L, Bergh J, et al. 10-Year results after sector resection with or without postoperative radiotherapy for stage I breast cancer: a randomized trial. J Clin Oncol 1999;17(8):2326–33.

17. Renton SC, Gazet JC, Ford HT, et al. The importance of the resection margin in conservative surgery for breast cancer. Eur J Surg Oncol 1996;22(1):17–22.

18. Clark RM, Whelan T, Levine M, et al. Randomized clinical trial of breast irradiation following lumpectomy and axillary dissection for node-negative breast cancer: an update. Ontario Clinical Oncology Group. J Natl Cancer Inst 1996;88(22):1659–64.

19. Forrest AP, Stewart HJ, Everington D, et al. Randomised controlled trial of conservation therapy for breast cancer: 6-year analysis of the Scottish trial. Scottish Cancer Trials Breast Group. Lancet 1996;348(9029):708–13.

20. Veronesi U, Marubini E, Mariani L, et al. Radiotherapy after breast-conserving surgery in small breast carcinoma: long-term results of a randomized trial. Ann Oncol 2001;12(7):997–1003.

21. Fisher B, Bryant J, Dignam JJ, et al. Tamoxifen, radiation therapy, or both for prevention of ipsilateral breast tumor recurrence after lumpectomy in women with invasive breast cancers of one centimeter or less. J Clin Oncol 2002;20(20):4141–9.

22. Fyles AW, McCready DR, Manchul LA, et al. Tamoxifen with or without breast irradiation in women 50 years of age or older with early breast cancer. N Engl J Med 2004;351(10):963–70.

23. Hughes KS, Schnaper LA, Berry D, et al. Lumpectomy plus tamoxifen with or without irradiation in women 70 years of age or older with early breast cancer. N Engl J Med 2004;351(10):971–7.

24. Fisher B, Dignam J, Wolmark N, et al. Tamoxifen and chemotherapy for lymph node-negative, estrogen receptor-positive breast cancer. J Natl Cancer Inst 1997;89(22):1673–82.

25. Arriagada R, Spielmann M, Koscielny S, et al. Patterns of failure in a randomized trial of adjuvant chemotherapy in postmenopausal patients with early breast cancer treated with tamoxifen. Ann Oncol 2002;13(9):1378–86.

26. Krag DN, Anderson SJ, Julian TB, et al. Technical outcomes of sentinel-lymph-node resection and conventional axillary-lymph-node dissection in patients with clinically node-negative breast cancer: results from the NSABP B-32 randomised phase III trial. Lancet Oncol 2007;8(10):881–8.

27. Krag DN, Anderson SJ, Julian TB, et al. Sentinel-lymph-node resection compared with conventional axillary-lymph-node dissection in clinically node-negative patients with breast cancer: overall survival findings from the NSABP B-32 randomised phase 3 trial. Lancet Oncol 2010;11(10):927–33.

28. Zavagno G, De Salvo GL, Scalco G, et al. A randomized clinical trial on sentinel lymph node biopsy versus axillary lymph node dissection in breast cancer: results of the Sentinella/GIVOM trial. Ann Surg 2008;247(2):207–13.

29. Ashikaga T, Krag DN, Land SR, et al. Morbidity results from the NSABP B-32 trial comparing sentinel lymph node dissection versus axillary dissection. J Surg Oncol 2010;102(2):111–8.

30. Mansel RE, Fallowfield L, Kissin M, et al. Randomized multicenter trial of sentinel node biopsy versus standard axillary treatment in operable breast cancer: the ALMANAC Trial. J Natl Cancer Inst 2006;98(9):599–609.

31. Veronesi U, Paganelli G, Viale G, et al. Sentinel-lymph-node biopsy as a staging procedure in breast cancer: update of a randomised controlled study. Lancet Oncol 2006;7(12):983–90.

32. Giuliano AE, Hunt KK, Ballman KV, et al. Axillary dissection vs no axillary dissection in women with invasive breast cancer and sentinel node metastasis: a randomized clinical trial. JAMA 2011;305(6):569–75.

33. Fisher B, Bryant J, Wolmark N, et al. Effect of preoperative chemotherapy on the outcome of women with operable breast cancer. J Clin Oncol 1998;16(8):2672–85.

34. Rastogi P, Anderson SJ, Bear HD, et al. Preoperative chemotherapy: updates of National Surgical Adjuvant Breast and Bowel Project protocols B-18 and B-27. J Clin Oncol 2008;26(5):778–85.

35. Ellis MJ, Suman VJ, Hoog J, et al. Randomized phase II neoadjuvant comparison between letrozole, anastrozole, and exemestane for postmenopausal women with estrogen receptor-rich stage 2 to 3 breast cancer: clinical and biomarker outcomes and predictive value of the baseline PAM50-based intrinsic subtype– ACOSOG Z1031. J Clin Oncol 2011;29(17):2342–9.

36. Paik S, Shak S, Tang G, et al. A multigene assay to predict recurrence of tamoxifen-treated, node-negative breast cancer. N Engl J Med 2004;351(27):2817–26.

37. Miles W. A method of performing abdominoperineal excision for carcinoma of the rectum and the terminal portion of the pelvic colon. Lancet 1908;2:1812–3.

38. Dixon CF. Anterior resection for malignant lesions of the upper part of the rectum and lower part of the sigmoid. Ann Surg 1948;128(3):425–42.

39. Williams NS, Dixon MF, Johnston D. Reappraisal of the 5 centimetre rule of distal excision for carcinoma of the rectum: a study of distal intramural spread and of patients' survival. Br J Surg 1983;70(3):150–4.

40. Fisher B, Wolmark N, Rockette H, et al. Postoperative adjuvant chemotherapy or radiation therapy for rectal cancer: results from NSABP protocol R-01. J Natl Cancer Inst 1988;80(1):21–9.

41. Randomised trial of surgery alone versus surgery followed by radiotherapy for mobile cancer of the rectum. Medical Research Council Rectal Cancer Working Party. Lancet 1996;348(9042):1610–4.

42. Wolmark N, Wieand HS, Hyams DM, et al. Randomized trial of postoperative adjuvant chemotherapy with or without radiotherapy for carcinoma of the rectum: National Surgical Adjuvant Breast and Bowel Project Protocol R-02. J Natl Cancer Inst 2000;92(5):388–96.

43. Bentzen SM, Balslev I, Pedersen M, et al. Time to loco-regional recurrence after resection of Dukes' B and C colorectal cancer with or without adjuvant postoperative radiotherapy. A multivariate regression analysis. Br J Cancer 1992;65(1):102–7.

44. Prolongation of the disease-free interval in surgically treated rectal carcinoma. Gastrointestinal Tumor Study Group. N Engl J Med 1985;312(23):1465–72.
45. Douglass HO Jr, Moertel CG, Mayer RJ, et al. Survival after postoperative combination treatment of rectal cancer. N Engl J Med 1986;315(20):1294–5.
46. Adjuvant radiotherapy for rectal cancer: a systematic overview of 8,507 patients from 22 randomised trials. Lancet 2001;358(9290):1291–304.
47. Krook JE, Moertel CG, Gunderson LL, et al. Effective surgical adjuvant therapy for high-risk rectal carcinoma. N Engl J Med 1991;324(11):709–15.
48. Adjuvant therapy for patients with colon and rectum cancer. Consens Statement 1990;8(4):1–25.
49. Gerard A, Buyse M, Nordlinger B, et al. Preoperative radiotherapy as adjuvant treatment in rectal cancer. Final results of a randomized study of the European Organization for Research and Treatment of Cancer (EORTC). Ann Surg 1988;208(5):606–14.
50. Cedermark B, Johansson H, Rutqvist LE, et al. The Stockholm I trial of preoperative short term radiotherapy in operable rectal carcinoma. A prospective randomized trial. Stockholm Colorectal Cancer Study Group. Cancer 1995; 75(9):2269–75.
51. Randomized study on preoperative radiotherapy in rectal carcinoma. Stockholm Colorectal Cancer Study Group. Ann Surg Oncol 1996;3(5):423–30.
52. Folkesson J, Birgisson H, Pahlman L, et al. Swedish Rectal Cancer Trial: long lasting benefits from radiotherapy on survival and local recurrence rate. J Clin Oncol 2005;23(24):5644–50.
53. Birgisson H, Pahlman L, Gunnarsson U, et al. Late gastrointestinal disorders after rectal cancer surgery with and without preoperative radiation therapy. Br J Surg 2008;95(2):206–13.
54. Sebag-Montefiore D, Stephens RJ, Steele R, et al. Preoperative radiotherapy versus selective postoperative chemoradiotherapy in patients with rectal cancer (MRC CR07 and NCIC-CTG C016): a multicentre, randomised trial. Lancet 2009; 373(9666):811–20.
55. Sauer R, Becker H, Hohenberger W, et al. Preoperative versus postoperative chemoradiotherapy for rectal cancer. N Engl J Med 2004;351(17):1731–40.
56. Roh MS, Colangelo LH, O'Connell MJ, et al. Preoperative multimodality therapy improves disease-free survival in patients with carcinoma of the rectum: NSABP R-03. J Clin Oncol 2009;27(31):5124–30.
57. Dahl O, Horn A, Morild I, et al. Low-dose preoperative radiation postpones recurrences in operable rectal cancer. Results of a randomized multicenter trial in western Norway. Cancer 1990;66(11):2286–94.
58. Camma C, Giunta M, Fiorica F, et al. Preoperative radiotherapy for resectable rectal cancer: a meta-analysis. JAMA 2000;284(8):1008–15.
59. Kapiteijn E, Marijnen CA, Nagtegaal ID, et al. Preoperative radiotherapy combined with total mesorectal excision for resectable rectal cancer. N Engl J Med 2001;345(9):638–46.
60. Peeters KC, Marijnen CA, Nagtegaal ID, et al. The TME trial after a median follow-up of 6 years: increased local control but no survival benefit in irradiated patients with resectable rectal carcinoma. Ann Surg 2007;246(5):693–701.
61. van Gijn W, Marijnen CA, Nagtegaal ID, et al. Preoperative radiotherapy combined with total mesorectal excision for resectable rectal cancer: 12-year follow-up of the multicentre, randomised controlled TME trial. Lancet Oncol 2011;12(6):575–82.
62. Bosset JF, Collette L, Calais G, et al. Chemotherapy with preoperative radiotherapy in rectal cancer. N Engl J Med 2006;355(11):1114–23.

63. Bujko K, Nowacki MP, Nasierowska-Guttmejer A, et al. Long-term results of a randomized trial comparing preoperative short-course radiotherapy with preoperative conventionally fractionated chemoradiation for rectal cancer. Br J Surg 2006;93(10):1215–23.

64. Gerard JP, Conroy T, Bonnetain F, et al. Preoperative radiotherapy with or without concurrent fluorouracil and leucovorin in T3-4 rectal cancers: results of FFCD 9203. J Clin Oncol 2006;24(28):4620–5.

65. Latkauskas T, Paskauskas S, Dambrauskas Z, et al. Preoperative chemoradiation vs radiation alone for stage II and III resectable rectal cancer: a meta-analysis. Colorectal Dis 2010;12(11):1075–83.

66. Bujko K, Glynne-Jones R, Bujko M. Does adjuvant fluoropyrimidine-based chemotherapy provide a benefit for patients with resected rectal cancer who have already received neoadjuvant radiochemotherapy? A systematic review of randomised trials. Ann Oncol 2010;21(9):1743–50.

67. Nelson H, Petrelli N, Carlin A, et al. Guidelines 2000 for colon and rectal cancer surgery. J Natl Cancer Inst 2001;93(8):583–96.

68. Jayne DG, Thorpe HC, Copeland J, et al. Five-year follow-up of the Medical Research Council CLASICC trial of laparoscopically assisted versus open surgery for colorectal cancer. Br J Surg 2010;97(11):1638–45.

69. Guillou PJ, Quirke P, Thorpe H, et al. Short-term endpoints of conventional versus laparoscopic-assisted surgery in patients with colorectal cancer (MRC CLASICC trial): multicentre, randomised controlled trial. Lancet 2005;365(9472):1718–26.

70. Jayne DG, Guillou PJ, Thorpe H, et al. Randomized trial of laparoscopic-assisted resection of colorectal carcinoma: 3-year results of the UK MRC CLASICC Trial Group. J Clin Oncol 2007;25(21):3061–8.

71. Lujan J, Valero G, Hernandez Q, et al. Randomized clinical trial comparing laparoscopic and open surgery in patients with rectal cancer. Br J Surg 2009;96(9):982–9.

72. Lezoche G, Baldarelli M, Guerrieri M, et al. A prospective randomized study with a 5-year minimum follow-up evaluation of transanal endoscopic microsurgery versus laparoscopic total mesorectal excision after neoadjuvant therapy. Surg Endosc 2008;22(2):352–8.

73. Winde G, Nottberg H, Keller R, et al. Surgical cure for early rectal carcinomas (T1). Transanal endoscopic microsurgery vs. anterior resection. Dis Colon Rectum 1996;39(9):969–76.

74. Paty PB, Nash GM, Baron P, et al. Long-term results of local excision for rectal cancer. Ann Surg 2002;236(4):522–9 [discussion: 529–30].

75. Mellgren A, Sirivongs P, Rothenberger DA, et al. Is local excision adequate therapy for early rectal cancer? Dis Colon Rectum 2000;43(8):1064–71 [discussion: 1071–4].

76. You YN, Baxter NN, Stewart A, et al. Is the increasing rate of local excision for stage I rectal cancer in the United States justified? A nationwide cohort study from the National Cancer Database. Ann Surg 2007;245(5):726–33.

77. Sachdeva AK, Russell TR. Safe introduction of new procedures and emerging technologies in surgery: education, credentialing, and privileging. Surg Clin North Am 2007;87(4):853–66, vi–vii.

78. Krag D, Weaver D, Ashikaga T, et al. The sentinel node in breast cancer–a multi-center validation study. N Engl J Med 1998;339(14):941–6.

79. Tafra L, McMasters KM, Whitworth P, et al. Credentialing issues with sentinel lymph node staging for breast cancer. Am J Surg 2000;180(4):268–73.

80. McMasters KM, Wong SL, Chao C, et al. Defining the optimal surgeon experience for breast cancer sentinel lymph node biopsy: a model for implementation of new surgical techniques. Ann Surg 2001;234(3):292–9 [discussion: 299–300].

81. Harlow SP, Krag DN, Julian TB, et al. Prerandomization Surgical Training for the National Surgical Adjuvant Breast and Bowel Project (NSABP) B-32 trial: a randomized phase III clinical trial to compare sentinel node resection to conventional axillary dissection in clinically node-negative breast cancer. Ann Surg 2005;241(1):48–54.
82. Barker AD, Sigman CC, Kelloff GJ, et al. I-SPY 2: an adaptive breast cancer trial design in the setting of neoadjuvant chemotherapy. Clin Pharmacol Ther 2009; 86(1):97–100.
83. American College of Surgeons accredited education institutes. 2011. Available at: http://www.facs.org/education/accreditationprogram/. Accessed November 2, 2011.
84. Merkow RP, Ko CY. Evidence-based medicine in surgery: the importance of both experimental and observational study designs. JAMA 2011;306(4):436–7.

Patient Safety in Surgical Oncology

Perspective From the Operating Room

Yue-Yung Hu, MD, MPH[a,b], Caprice C. Greenberg, MD, MPH[c],*

KEYWORDS

- Safety • Operating room • Human factors • Error

KEY POINTS

- Human factors engineering is a methodology well suited for the study of complex intra-operative processes.
- Video provides a promising means of studying human factors in the OR.
- Providers are predisposed to committing active errors through latent conditions in the system.
- Adaptability is a positive aspect of human variability that constitutes the last line of defense against error.

INTRODUCTION

In 1999, the Institute of Medicine[1] published "To Err is Human: Building a Safer Health Care System," emphasizing the prevalence of preventable medical errors in American health care and the role of systems, processes, and conditions in ensuring (or undermining) safety. Because 50% to 65% of inpatient adverse events are experienced by surgical patients,[2] and 75% of these occur intraoperatively,[3] the operating room (OR) is a high-impact area for safety improvements.

Traditionally, surgical vulnerability has been measured in terms of preoperative risk (patient and procedural risk factors,[4] surgeon volume,[5] and institutional volume),[6] whereas safety has been defined by the absence of postoperative morbidity or mortality. The intraoperative phase of care, despite its obvious relevance to the field of surgical safety and rich potential as a data source, has been largely neglected.

The authors have nothing to disclose.

[a] Department of Surgery, Center for Surgery & Public Health, Brigham & Women's Hospital, One Brigham Circle, 1620 Tremont Street, Suite 4-020, Boston, MA 02115, USA; [b] Department of Surgery, Beth Israel Deaconess Medical Center, 110 Francis Street, Suite 9B, Boston, MA 02215, USA; [c] Wisconsin Surgical Outcomes Research Program, Department of Surgery, University of Wisconsin Hospitals & Clinics, 600 Highland Avenue H4/730, Madison, WI 53792-7375, USA
* Corresponding author.
E-mail address: greenberg@surgery.wisc.edu

Because it is understudied, many gaps exist in our knowledge of the intraoperative factors that contribute to or detract from patient safety. Therefore, few evidence-based guidelines or interventions exist to support hospitals or their providers in the OR.[7–10]

Surgery is an inherently hazardous work domain requiring high reliability. Safe operations result from the successful coordination of individuals and teams of diverse training and experience levels, working within complex hospital systems, under constraints imposed by time, uncertainty, and health status. Human factors engineering, focusing on "the interaction among humans and other elements of a system…physical, cognitive, organizational, environmental, and other,"[11] has been deployed and is responsible for safety and reliability advances in other, similarly high-risk industries, such as aeronautics or nuclear reactor control. Addressing the origins of error at all levels—individual, team, and system—human factors analysis is an ideal tool for the study of safety in the OR.

THEORETICAL MODELS
Error

In his 1990 treatise, "Human Error," Jim Reason[12] describes his Swiss cheese model of error (**Fig. 1**). In it, the system is represented by a stack of Swiss cheese slices, each analogous to a protective layer in the system, with holes symbolizing the potential for failure at each step in the process. Because the holes in Swiss cheese (the vulnerabilities of a system) are not continuous throughout a stack (the system), most problems are stopped at one layer or another, before they culminate in a larger, more consequential error. For a catastrophic failure to occur, the holes must be aligned at every level.

As per Reason, these holes may be of two types: active and latent. Active errors are those that are traditionally invoked during discussions about adverse events: readily apparent, they are committed by a human at "the sharp end," or at the point of care. A retained foreign body, for example, represents an active error: the failure to remove an instrument at the end of an operation. However, humans do not make these errors in isolation; they are predisposed toward them by latent conditions at "the blunt end," in the system. Leaving an instrument in a patient is not the act of an individual surgeon. Rather, it is one precipitated by existing flaws in the organizational design of the entire process: the cumbersome and error-prone nature of the counting protocol, for example.[13,14]

Resilience

In recent years, human factors experts have begun to view the human as the hero rather than the source of error. In his follow-up book, "The Human Contribution,"

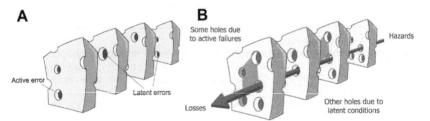

Fig. 1. Reason's Swiss Cheese Model of Error. (*A*) Each slice of cheese represents a barrier in the system. The holes in each slice represent opportunities for failure at each step, active or latent. (*B*) Alignment of the system's vulnerabilities allows "hazards" to become "losses," or smaller errors to culminate in a larger, more consequential one. (*From* Reason JT. The human contribution. Farnham, Surrey, England: Ashgate Publishing Limited; 2008; with permission.)

Reason[15] cautions against "an excessive reliance on system measures," because it is individuals that constitute a system's last line of defense against error. With the uniquely human ability to anticipate and adapt to changing circumstances, people are capable of recovering problems that have managed to propagate through even the most thoughtfully designed systems. This heroism, however, has its limits. Citing Carthey and colleagues'[16] observational study of arterial switch operations, in which an increased risk of death was demonstrated with higher numbers of minor events regardless of compensation, Reason proposes a knotted rubber band model of system resilience (**Fig. 2**). In it, the system is analogous to a rubber band, with a knot in the middle to represent current operating conditions. To maintain safety, the knot must stay within a narrow operating zone; stretch applied in one direction by dangerous perturbations in the system must be counteracted by compensatory corrections in the opposite direction. With a rising number of perturbations and corrections, the system becomes distorted beyond its capacity to respond.

METHODOLOGIES
Retrospective Studies

The characterization of intraoperative human and system factors that impact safety has thus far been limited. Among available methodologies, the most widely used is the retrospective reconstruction of the intraoperative events: root or common cause analysis,[17,18] for example, or the analysis of malpractice claims data.[3,19,20] Although this research has been informative about the specific factors that may lead to adverse outcomes, it is susceptible to bias.[21] These post hoc analyses suffer from inaccurate or incomplete recall; without a contemporaneous record, it is difficult to capture all of the mechanisms that have culminated in error. Furthermore, focusing research efforts on the negative effects of care selects for only part of all the available data; information regarding events that are averted or compensated, processes that would be highly instructive in understanding safety in the OR, is lost.

Field Observations

Prospective data collection in the OR, therefore, is needed to completely describe the intraoperative delivery of care. Field observations have been described by several

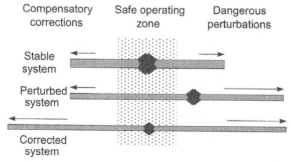

Fig. 2. Reason's Knotted Rubber Band Model of System Resilience. The rubber band represents the system, and the knot represents current operating conditions. To maintain safety, the knot must remain in the "safe operating zone" (*dotted area*). Dangerous perturbations in one direction may pull the current operating conditions out of the safe zone (*second rubber band*). To re-establish safety, compensatory corrections must be applied in the other direction (*third rubber band*). The system has a maximum capacity for stretch. (*From* Reason JT. The human contribution. Farnham, Surrey, England: Ashgate Publishing Limited; 2008; with permission.)

groups[14,16,22–33] but have yet to be broadly applied; most of these studies are restricted to small case series at single institutions, for several reasons. First, human factors engineering is a new field to medicine, and few people with experience in both disciplines (or multidisciplinary collaborations) exist. Access to the OR may be difficult to attain because of an underrecognition of intraoperative safety problems and cultural mores regarding provider privacy in the workplace. Those who are successful in gaining entry are likely to encounter additional cognitive barriers to the complete transcription of intraoperative events; it can be difficult to completely observe multiple simultaneous conversations or incidents, to link all downstream occurrences to all earlier preconditions, and to recall everything after the surgery has ended. Moreover, because only a few extra people may unobtrusively be present in any OR at one time, the comprehension of ongoing events may only be as complete as the knowledge base or memory of the observers; consultation with domain experts for clarification purposes may only be realized retrospectively. Nevertheless, most evidence about human factors in the OR has been generated using live field observations and will be reviewed.

Video-Based Observations

In circumventing many of the aforementioned methodological limitations, video-based analyses[34,35] hold great potential for furthering the study of safety in the OR. Video may be recorded prospectively but reviewed retrospectively and repeatedly, until all events are fully understood and the connections between them are completely deciphered. Therefore, it eliminates many of the issues surrounding observer recall and subjectivity. Additionally, it may serve as an educational tool, a mechanism for providing targeted feedback to individuals, teams, and organizational leaders. However, video poses its own challenges. Although it is theoretically indiscriminate in its capture, it may still generate incomplete data, depending on the technologic capacity or functionality of the audiovisual equipment. Additionally, providers may be reluctant to be recorded because of fears that the recordings will be used during performance evaluations[36] or in courts of law.[35] These concerns may be addressed, at least partly, by carefully constructing research protocols with multiple layers of protection for study subjects, including restricted data access, scheduled data destruction, and acquisition of a Certificate of Confidentiality.[37] This article reviews the evidence generated using video in the OR.

HUMAN FACTORS IN THE OR

For the purposes of this discussion, human factors are divided into those pertaining to humans and those corresponding to the system. Human attributes are relevant to performance both individually and within a team, and include qualities such as communication, coordination, cooperation, leadership, and vigilance. System features circumscribe the environment in which humans work, for example the equipment they use, the structure of the larger organization in which they work, or the policies that govern them. Several examples from the literature are detailed here. These examples are intended to be illustrative only; they are not exhaustive lists of human factors.

Humans

As active errors were originally conceived by Reason, human cognitive limitations were the most proximal causal factor. The imperfect behavior of individuals, it was thought, makes them prone to failures at all stages of performance: planning (mistakes, ie, flawed intentions), memory storage (lapses, ie, omissions), and task execution (slips, ie, failure to act as planned). Although humans are now viewed with increasing positivity, as agents of recovery, rather than sources of erraticism, their abilities are still subject to limitations. Although individuals are recognized for their ability to compensate, this capacity diminishes with progressive perturbations in the system. The most competent nurse can slip when counting, and is even more likely to do so if simultaneously juggling the surgeons' requests for new instruments and the anesthesiologists' need for blood products, coordinating with the preoperative and postoperative units, and answering the resident's pager. In the past, human limitations have been countered with increased standardization, based upon the theory that these additional barriers to atypical behavior would protect against failure. Protocols requiring radiographs or automating the count procedure with bar-coding[7] or radiofrequency identification technology[38] decrease reliance on the error-prone manual count. However, recent human factors data indicate that flexibility is needed in the system to permit heroes to maneuver[39]; one must remain cognizant of the fact that even well-intended protocols (like the manual count) run the risk of inadvertently disabling providers.[13] An appropriate balance between minimizing human slips, lapses, and mistakes and maximizing human heroic potential must be maintained.

Communication is one of the most studied and most critical human factors in medicine. Root cause analyses of sentinel events reported to the Joint Commission from 2004 through 2011 implicate faulty communication in 56% of operative or postoperative complications, 64% of retained foreign bodies, and 69% of wrong patient, wrong site, or wrong procedure cases.[40] The importance of communication is further supported by reviews of surgical malpractice claims. Griffen and colleagues[41] attribute 22% of complications to miscommunication, making it the most pervasive behavioral problem of all they investigated, whereas Greenberg and colleagues[19] place 30% of all communication breakdowns in the OR. Lingard and colleagues[42] estimate that 31% of all procedurally relevant communications in the OR fail; of these, 36% have tangible effects, such as inefficiency, delay, resource waste, or procedural error.

Miscommunication has multiple causes, and therefore is best addressed with a multipronged approach. Standardization may help in certain selected scenarios; protocols may serve as memory aids, for example, ensuring that all salient points are covered in a discussion. After standardized communication was integrated into handoffs at Northwestern University,[43] surgical residents' perceptions of accuracy, completeness, and clarity during the transfer of care improved significantly. After implementing the Situation, Background, Assessment, and Recommendation model of communication into their surgical curriculum, a decrease in order entry errors was seen at the Mount Sinai School of Medicine.[44] The University of Washington's[45] computerized sign-out system allowed residents to spend more time with patients during prerounds and halved the number of patients missed on rounds, while improving resident ratings of continuity of care and workload.

Checklists work analogously in the OR, reminding providers to do the things that are relevant to almost every operation, but also have another important function. Unlike surgical inpatient teams, the OR team is multidisciplinary; the individuals that constitute it are more likely to differ in their understandings of the situation at hand. The checklist compels them to establish a shared mental model that enables each team member to better anticipate and plan his or her own role. Multinational studies have shown its impact on patient morbidity and mortality, as well as provider attitudes regarding safety.[9,46]

However, standardized protocols cannot help with most communication in the OR, such as that which occurs spontaneously, in response to continuously evolving events. In these situations, communication is best accomplished ad hoc, with flexibility for individuals to speak up about arising threats to safety as they see fit. To achieve safety, a level of candidness, and hence a sense of team is needed. The OR must be an environment in which each team member recognizes and is comfortable in his or her role as an equal contributor; it is therefore a form of checks and balances for each individual and the system. The importance of OR teamwork to patient outcomes is well established. Across 44 Veterans Affairs Medical centers and eight academic hospitals, OR team members who reported higher levels of positive communication and collaboration with attending and resident physicians on the surgical service were found to have lower risk-adjusted morbidity rates.[47] Mazzocco and colleagues[30] showed an increased odds of complications or death when intraoperative information sharing, a communication behavior that they distinguish from briefing and that incorporates "mutual respect" and "appropriate[ness]," was observed to be low. In Catchpole and colleagues'[26] observational study of laparoscopic cholecystectomies and carotid endarterectomies, higher leadership and management skills scores for surgeons and nurses correlated with shorter operating times and lower rates of procedural problems and errors outside the operating field, respectively.

As these studies show, a high degree of variability surrounds teamwork in the OR.[30,47] Even within a single OR team, the perception of it may differ, depending on the discipline of the reporting party.[48] Compared with anesthesiologists and nurses, surgeons seem to overestimate the communication and teamwork in the room.[49–51] These disparities may be the result of the traditional vertical hierarchy in surgery. Surgeons, at its top, are simply not the ones who feel constrained by it, and thus are less likely to recognize the value of a flattened one (ie, in the open communication or shared decision-making that it would promote).[51] Likewise, although nurses, anesthesiologists, and surgeons are equally capable of recognizing tension in the OR, they disagree on the responsibility for creating and resolving it.[52]

Although certainly more amorphous a target than a successful handoff or briefing, teamwork is amenable to intervention. After introducing a team training curriculum, Northwestern University[53] reduced their observable intraoperative communication failure rate from 0.7 per hour to 0.3 per hour. At the University of Oxford,[54] a nontechnical skills course decreased operative technical errors and nonoperative procedural errors during laparoscopic cholecystectomies. The Veterans Health Administration, having implemented a medical team training program for OR personnel in its facilities on a rolling basis, documented a decline in risk-adjusted surgical mortality rate that was 50% greater in the trained hospitals than in the untrained ones.[55] These interventions represent adaptations of Crew Resource Management (CRM), a training module developed in aviation to educate cockpit crews about communication (eg, assertiveness, briefing/debriefing), error management (eg, the recognition of "red flag" situations), and teamwork (eg, cross-checking, interpersonal skills, shared mental models, conflict resolution, and flat hierarchies),[54,56–58] and thus far have been conducted in a one-time fashion. Despite their apparent success, the investigators of these studies note the limitations of a single intervention; because the adoption of CRM techniques represents a significant cultural and professional shift in medicine, continuous training and feedback are needed.[54,56]

Several instruments have been developed for measuring teamwork in the OR, and may be considered for assessments of baseline needs, and measurements of postintervention change and sustainability over time. The Observational Teamwork Assessment for Surgery (OTAS) consists of a teamwork-related task checklist (patient tasks, equipment/provisions tasks, and communication tasks) and a global rating scale for teamwork-related behaviors (communication, coordination, leadership, monitoring, and cooperation). Although its developers report good interobserver reliability and content validity,[59] they have also described a learning curve for using it, which may limit its reproducibility by other groups.[60] The Oxford Non-Technical Skills System

(NOTECHS) rates each OR subteam (anesthesiology, nursing, surgery) on four dimensions: leadership and management; teamwork and cooperation; problem-solving and decision-making; and situation awareness. Its developers also have shown reliability and validity, and have correlated it with OTAS,[32] but it also has not found widespread use outside of its home institution.

The System

In an operation, the system may refer to the physical environment of that particular OR or the policies, practices, and organizational structure of the department or hospital. It may also implicate the professional culture or values of an institution as a whole, or that of the discipline of surgery.

As a human factor that describes the system, equipment has face validity for most surgeons; it is easy to appreciate the value in having functional, well-designed equipment available at the appropriate times. Healey and colleagues[61] documented 64 instances of unavailable or nonfunctional equipment in 35 of 50 observed general surgical procedures, and of all of the intraoperative distractions or interruption noted, these contributed the most to interference with the case. In 31 cardiac operations, Wiegmann and colleagues[24] mapped 11% of surgical flow disruptions ("deviations from the natural process of an operation") to difficulties with equipment or technology.

Perhaps less readily understood, but no less critical, are the organization processes of the OR. For example, in a traditional OR system, surgeons provides their own estimated case durations, a practice that introduces a great deal of subjectivity and variability, hindering attempts to match OR capacity to use. Without accurate approximations of case length, the appropriate allocation of human and equipment resources is difficult. The authors' own study[62] observed an instance in which more oncology cases were simultaneously booked than the number of oncology kits available; the team expended extra time and effort to obtain the necessary instruments in a piecemeal fashion, and the case was delayed. At the Mayo Clinic,[63] the development of a surgeon-specific procedural database to provide estimates for case duration based on historical and prospective moving averages was among several initiatives that led to increased OR efficiency and financial performance.

Similarly, in a traditional OR system, surgeons specify the contents of their own instrument kits. With this practice, thousands of case-cards or pick-tickets may result, consuming a significant amount of nursing and central processing time and effort. After nursing leadership and surgical faculty collaborated to consolidate and streamline the instrument trays at the University of Alabama,[64] tray and case cart errors decreased. Because circulators spent less time making phone calls to central sterile and flash-sterilizing instruments, their ability to attend to the case increased.

To the authors' knowledge, no instruments are available to assess the system in isolation. The Safety Attitudes Questionnaire[65] and the OR Management Attitudes Questionnaire[49] ask respondents to rate teamwork and describe the organizational climate toward safety. Wiegmann and colleagues'[24] system includes a teamwork category, and Healey and colleagues'[61] contains several measures of communication and "procedural" interference, as well as the environment. The Disruptions in Surgery Index also incorporates individual and team factors in its list of potential disruptions, and is essentially a survey, rather than an observational tool, querying respondents about the perceived impact on themselves and their team members.[66]

A CASE STUDY

The authors captured one particularly illustrative example on video in their own observational study.[62] During a procedure, an alarm began to sound, yet its source was unclear; the alert did not indicate to which piece of equipment it belonged, nor whether it represented equipment malfunction or patient endangerment. As the surgeons continued to operate, the nurses and anesthesiologists became absorbed in its investigation. After several minutes, the circulator took charge of the situation, sent the anesthesiologists back to the head of the bed, and called biomedical engineering for help. Eventually, a failed warmer was determined to be the source, and a new one was brought.

Because nothing adverse happened, this incident would likely have been dismissed, rather than reported. However, it provides useful information. An analogous case in the aviation industry, in which recovery was not achieved, warns against ignoring these data. In 1974, the landing gear indicator light on Eastern Airlines Flight 401 failed to illuminate. While the crew preoccupied itself with troubleshooting the issue, the autopilot became deactivated and the flight crashed.[67] The tragedy of the event lies in the fact that the landing gear could have been lowered manually; 101 people died as a result of a burned-out lightbulb (equipment that was unimportant to the flight) and a failure of the team to maintain situational awareness (vigilance) and manage their human resources (delegate the responsibilities for troubleshooting and flying to separate people).

The authors' case displayed similar equipment problems (malfunction and poor design), and an initial failure of the team to maintain situational awareness and manage their human resources. However, the smooth engagement of team—leadership of the circulator and cooperation from the anesthesiologists and the biomedical engineers—led to a quick recovery, and may have prevented the occurrence of a more catastrophic event.

SUMMARY

In the OR, as in other high-acuity, high-reliability work environments, human and system factors interact to impact safety. The complex interrelations and interdependencies among people, resources, information, and technology must be more clearly delineated if successful interventions are to be developed. The authors emphasize that success must not be determined narrowly; given the intricate interconnections between various human factors in the OR and the importance of flexibility to system resilience, all consequences must be evaluated. Emerging techniques for conducting this research hold much promise in the advancement of the understanding of intraoperative safety.

REFERENCES

1. Kohn LT, Corrigan JM, Donaldson MS. To err is human: building a safer health system. Institute of Medicine. Washington, DC: National Academy Press; 2000.
2. Gawande AA, Thomas EJ, Zinner MJ, et al. The incidence and nature of surgical adverse events in Colorado and Utah in 1992. Surgery 1999;126(1):66–75.
3. Rogers SO Jr, Gawande AA, Kwaan M, et al. Analysis of surgical errors in closed malpractice claims at 4 liability insurers. Surgery 2006;140(1):25–33.
4. Raval MV, Cohen ME, Ingraham AM, et al. Improving American College of Surgeons National Surgical Quality Improvement Program risk adjustment: incorporation of a novel procedure risk score. J Am Coll Surg 2010;211(6):715–23.
5. Birkmeyer JD, Stukel TA, Siewers AE, et al. Surgeon volume and operative mortality in the United States. N Engl J Med 2003;349(22):2117–27.

6. Birkmeyer JD, Dimick JB, Staiger DO. Operative mortality and procedure volume as predictors of subsequent hospital performance. Ann Surg 2006;243(3): 411–7.

7. Greenberg CC, Diaz-Flores R, Lipsitz SR, et al. Bar-coding surgical sponges to improve safety: a randomized controlled trial. Ann Surg 2008;247(4):612–6.

8. Lingard L, Regehr G, Orser B, et al. Evaluation of a preoperative checklist and team briefing among surgeons, nurses, and anesthesiologists to reduce failures in communication. Arch Surg 2008;143(1):12–7 [discussion: 18].

9. Haynes AB, Weiser TG, Berry WR, et al. A surgical safety checklist to reduce morbidity and mortality in a global population. N Engl J Med 2009;360(5): 491–9.

10. Michaels RK, Makary MA, Dahab Y, et al. Achieving the National Quality Forum's "Never Events": prevention of wrong site, wrong procedure, and wrong patient operations. Ann Surg 2007;245(4):526–32.

11. International Ergonomics Association. What is ergonomics? Available at: http://www.iea.cc/browse.php?contID=what_is_ergonomics. Accessed April 6, 2010.

12. Reason JT. Human error. 1st edition. Cambridge (UK): Cambridge University Press; 1990.

13. Dierks MM, Christian CK, Roth EM. Healthcare safety: the impact of disabling safety protocols. IEEE Transactions on Systems, Man, and Cybernetics Part A: Systems and Humans 2004;34(6):693–8.

14. Christian CK, Gustafson ML, Roth EM, et al. A prospective study of patient safety in the operating room. Surgery 2006;139(2):159–73.

15. Reason JT. The human contribution. 1st edition. Farnham, Surrey, England: Ashgate Publishing, Limited; 2008.

16. Carthey J, de Leval MR, Reason JT. The human factor in cardiac surgery: errors and near misses in a high technology medical domain. Ann Thorac Surg 2001; 72(1):300–5.

17. Mallett R, Conroy M, Saslaw LZ, et al. Preventing wrong site, procedure, and patient events using a common cause analysis. Am J Med Qual 2012;27(1):21–9.

18. Faltz LL, Morley JN, Flink E, et al. The New York model: root cause analysis driving patient safety initiative to ensure correct surgical and invasive procedures. In: Henriksen K, Battles JB, Keyes MA, et al, editors. Advances in Patient Safety: New Directions and Alternative Approaches (Vol. 1: Assessment). Rockville (MD): Agency for Healthcare Research and Qaulity; 2008.

19. Greenberg CC, Regenbogen SE, Studdert DM, et al. Patterns of communication breakdowns resulting in injury to surgical patients. J Am Coll Surg 2007;204(4): 533–40.

20. Regenbogen SE, Greenberg CC, Studdert DM, et al. Patterns of technical error among surgical malpractice claims: an analysis of strategies to prevent injury to surgical patients. Ann Surg 2007;246(5):705–11.

21. Gopher D. Why it is not sufficient to study errors and incidents: human factors and safety in medical systems. Biomed Instrum Technol 2004;38(5):387–91.

22. Roth EM, Christian CK, Gustafson ML, et al. Using field observations as a tool for discovery: analysing cognitive and collaborative demands in the operating room. Cognit Tech Work 2004;6:148–57.

23. Schraagen JM, Schouten T, Smit M, et al. Assessing and improving teamwork in cardiac surgery. Qual Saf Health Care 2010;19(6):e29.

24. Wiegmann DA, ElBardissi AW, Dearani JA, et al. Disruptions in surgical flow and their relationship to surgical errors: an exploratory investigation. Surgery 2007; 142(5):658–65.

25. Arora S, Hull L, Sevdalis N, et al. Factors compromising safety in surgery: stressful events in the operating room. Am J Surg 2010;199(1):60–5.
26. Catchpole K, Mishra A, Handa A, et al. Teamwork and error in the operating room: analysis of skills and roles. Ann Surg 2008;247(4):699–706.
27. de Leval MR, Carthey J, Wright DJ, et al. Human factors and cardiac surgery: a multicenter study. J Thorac Cardiovasc Surg 2000;119(4 Pt 1):661–72.
28. Healey AN, Undre S, Vincent CA. Developing observational measures of performance in surgical teams. Qual Saf Health Care 2004;13(Suppl 1):i33–40.
29. Lingard L, Reznick R, Espin S, et al. Team communications in the operating room: talk patterns, sites of tension, and implications for novices. Acad Med 2002;77(3): 232–7.
30. Mazzocco K, Petitti DB, Fong KT, et al. Surgical team behaviors and patient outcomes. Am J Surg 2009;197(5):678–85.
31. Mishra A, Catchpole K, Dale T, et al. The influence of non-technical performance on technical outcome in laparoscopic cholecystectomy. Surg Endosc 2008;22(1): 68–73.
32. Mishra A, Catchpole K, McCulloch P. The Oxford NOTECHS System: reliability and validity of a tool for measuring teamwork behaviour in the operating theatre. Qual Saf Health Care 2009;18(2):104–8.
33. Parker SE, Laviana AA, Wadhera RK, et al. Development and evaluation of an observational tool for assessing surgical flow disruptions and their impact on surgical performance. World J Surg 2010;34(2):353–61.
34. Guerlain S, Adams RB, Turrentine FB, et al. Assessing team performance in the operating room: development and use of a "black-box" recorder and other tools for the intraoperative environment. J Am Coll Surg 2005;200(1):29–37.
35. Xiao Y, Schimpff S, Mackenzie C, et al. Video technology to advance safety in the operating room and perioperative environment. Surg Innov 2007;14(1):52–61.
36. Kim YJ, Xiao Y, Hu P, et al. Staff acceptance of video monitoring for coordination: a video system to support perioperative situation awareness. J Clin Nurs 2009; 18(16):2366–71.
37. Guerlain S, Turrentine B, Adams R, et al. Using video data for the analysis and training of medical personnel. Cognit Tech Work 2004;6:131–8.
38. Macario A, Morris D, Morris S. Initial clinical evaluation of a handheld device for detecting retained surgical gauze sponges using radiofrequency identification technology. Arch Surg 2006;141(7):659–62.
39. Sheridan TB. Risk, human error, and system resilience: fundamental ideas. Hum Factors 2008;50(3):418–26.
40. The Joint Commission. Sentinel event data: root causes by event type 2004-2011. In: Sentinel Event - Statistics. Available at: http://www.jointcommission.org/assets/ 1/18/Root_Causes_Event_Type_2004-2011.pdf. Accessed April 10, 2012.
41. Griffen FD, Stephens LS, Alexander JB, et al. Violations of behavioral practices revealed in closed claims reviews. Ann Surg 2008;248(3):468–74.
42. Lingard L, Espin S, Whyte S, et al. Communication failures in the operating room: an observational classification of recurrent types and effects. Qual Saf Health Care 2004;13(5):330–4.
43. Wayne JD, Tyagi R, Reinhardt G, et al. Simple standardized patient handoff system that increases accuracy and completeness. J Surg Educ 2008;65(6): 476–85.
44. Telem DA, Buch KE, Ellis S, et al. Integration of a formalized handoff system into the surgical curriculum: resident perspectives and early results. Arch Surg 2011; 146(1):89–93.

45. Van Eaton EG, Horvath KD, Lober WB, et al. A randomized, controlled trial evaluating the impact of a computerized rounding and sign-out system on continuity of care and resident work hours. J Am Coll Surg 2005;200(4):538–45.
46. Weiser TG, Haynes AB, Dziekan G, et al. Effect of a 19-item surgical safety checklist during urgent operations in a global patient population. Ann Surg 2010;251(5):976–80.
47. Davenport DL, Henderson WG, Mosca CL, et al. Risk-adjusted morbidity in teaching hospitals correlates with reported levels of communication and collaboration on surgical teams but not with scale measures of teamwork climate, safety climate, or working conditions. J Am Coll Surg 2007;205(6):778–84.
48. Makary MA, Sexton JB, Freischlag JA, et al. Operating room teamwork among physicians and nurses: teamwork in the eye of the beholder. J Am Coll Surg 2006;202(5):746–52.
49. Flin R, Yule S, McKenzie L, et al. Attitudes to teamwork and safety in the operating theatre. Surgeon 2006;4(3):145–51.
50. Mills P, Neily J, Dunn E. Teamwork and communication in surgical teams: implications for patient safety. J Am Coll Surg 2008;206(1):107–12.
51. Sexton JB, Thomas EJ, Helmreich RL. Error, stress, and teamwork in medicine and aviation: cross sectional surveys. BMJ 2000;320(7237):745–9.
52. Lingard L, Regehr G, Espin S, et al. Perceptions of operating room tension across professions: building generalizable evidence and educational resources. Acad Med 2005;80(Suppl 10):S75–9.
53. Halverson AL, Casey JT, Andersson J, et al. Communication failure in the operating room. Surgery 2011;149(3):305–10.
54. McCulloch P, Mishra A, Handa A, et al. The effects of aviation-style non-technical skills training on technical performance and outcome in the operating theatre. Qual Saf Health Care 2009;18(2):109–15.
55. Neily J, Mills PD, Young-Xu Y, et al. Association between implementation of a medical team training program and surgical mortality. JAMA 2010;304(15):1693–700.
56. Grogan EL, Stiles RA, France DJ, et al. The impact of aviation-based teamwork training on the attitudes of health-care professionals. J Am Coll Surg 2004; 199(6):843–8.
57. Hamman WR. The complexity of team training: what we have learned from aviation and its applications to medicine. Qual Saf Health Care 2004;13(Suppl 1):i72–9.
58. Burke CS, Salas E, Wilson-Donnelly K, et al. How to turn a team of experts into an expert medical team: guidance from the aviation and military communities. Qual Saf Health Care 2004;13(Suppl 1):i96–104.
59. Hull L, Arora S, Kassab E, et al. Observational teamwork assessment for surgery: content validation and tool refinement. J Am Coll Surg 2011;212(2):234–43, e231–5.
60. Sevdalis N, Lyons M, Healey AN, et al. Observational teamwork assessment for surgery: construct validation with expert versus novice raters. Ann Surg 2009; 249(6):1047–51.
61. Healey AN, Sevdalis N, Vincent CA. Measuring intra-operative interference from distraction and interruption observed in the operating theatre. Ergonomics 2006; 49(5–6):589–604.
62. Hu YY, Arriaga A, Roth EM, et al. Protecting patients from an unsafe system: the etiology and recovery of intra-operative deviations in care. Annals of Surgery 2012. In press.
63. Cima RR, Brown MJ, Hebl JR, et al. Use of lean six sigma methodology to improve operating room efficiency in a high-volume tertiary-care academic medical center. J Am Coll Surg 2011;213(1):83–92 [discussion: 93–4].

64. Heslin MJ, Doster BE, Daily SL, et al. Durable improvements in efficiency, safety, and satisfaction in the operating room. J Am Coll Surg 2008;206(5):1083–9 [discussion: 1089–90].
65. Sexton JB, Helmreich RL, Neilands TB, et al. The safety attitudes questionnaire: psychometric properties, benchmarking data, and emerging research. BMC Health Serv Res 2006;6:44.
66. Sevdalis N, Forrest D, Undre S, et al. Annoyances, disruptions, and interruptions in surgery: the Disruptions in Surgery Index (DiSI). World J Surg 2008;32(8): 1643–50.
67. Yanez L. Eastern flight 301: the story of the crash. Miami (FL): The Miami Herald; 2007.

Appropriate Use of Surgical Procedures for Patients with Cancer

Elise H. Lawson, MD, MSHS[a],[*],
Melinda Maggard Gibbons, MD, MSHS[a],
Clifford Y. Ko, MD, MS, MSHS[a],[b]

KEYWORDS

• Cancer • Appropriateness method • Surgery • Overuse • Underuse

KEY POINTS

- The appropriateness method was developed as a way to determine which patients should and should not undergo surgical intervention versus medical therapy.
- This method combines the best available evidence with expert opinion to produce explicit guidance on the risks and benefits of a procedure for specific indications.
- Overuse is generally defined as any instance in which a patient undergoes a procedure for an "inappropriate" indication.
- Underuse is generally defined as a patient with a "necessary" indication who does not receive the procedure.

Patients with cancer need a combination of life-saving and life-prolonging treatments, including systemic therapies, radiation, and surgical interventions. Providing high-quality cancer care means administering the right treatment, or combination of treatments, at the right time and in the correct way. Quality improvement efforts have generally focused on how care is given and on improving patient safety and reducing complications. Much less effort has been focused on ensuring that the correct treatments and procedures are selected for patients. For surgical oncology, this means determining whether or not surgery is indicated, when it should be performed relative to other treatments (such as neoadjuvant therapy), and which surgical procedure should be performed. A safe operation without any complications is not high-quality

[a] Department of Surgery, University of California, Los Angeles and VA Greater Los Angeles Healthcare System, 10833 LeConte Avenue, Los Angeles, CA 90095, USA; [b] Division of Research and Optimal Patient Care, American College of Surgeons, 633 North Saint Clair Street, Chicago, IL 60611, USA
* Corresponding author. Department of Surgery, UCLA Medical Center, CHS 72-215, 10833 LeConte Avenue, Los Angeles, CA 90095.
E-mail address: elawson@mednet.ucla.edu

Surg Oncol Clin N Am 21 (2012) 479–486
doi:10.1016/j.soc.2012.03.008
1055-3207/12/$ – see front matter © 2012 Elsevier Inc. All rights reserved.

care if a less invasive option is available or if the patient does not stand to benefit from the procedure. With the increasing focus on providing patient-centered care, it is time to ensure that patients with cancer are receiving treatments and surgical procedures that are not only safe and high quality, but also appropriate.

The appropriateness method was developed as a way to determine which patients should and should not undergo surgical intervention versus medical therapy. This method combines the best available evidence in the literature with expert opinion to produce explicit guidance for clinicians on the relative risks and benefits of a procedure for specific clinical indications.[1,2] Early research with this method focused on procedures, such as coronary artery bypass graft (CABG) surgery and carotid endarterectomy,[3] that have high associated morbidity and suspected inappropriate use. Subsequent studies focused on procedures such as colonoscopy,[3,4] hysterectomy,[5,6] bariatric surgery,[7] and cataract surgery,[8,9] among others.

Few appropriateness studies have focused on surgical oncology, likely because most patients with solid tumors routinely undergo surgery or are clearly not surgical candidates at the time of diagnosis (ie, stage 4). The appropriateness method, however, could also be used to determine the timing of surgical intervention for patients with cancer relative to other therapies and to compare the risks and benefits of surgical procedures with varying degrees of invasiveness. Because the method explicitly ranks the appropriateness of different treatment plans for a wide variety of clinical scenarios, it could help ensure that individual patients receive the best possible oncologic care.

Procedures chosen for study using the appropriateness method are generally those that are commonly performed, have elevated risk of morbidity and mortality, are controversial, and/or that use significant resources. A number of surgical oncology topics fit this description. For example, the appropriateness method could be used to explicitly divide patients with pancreatic cancer into 3 groups: those who would clearly benefit from surgery, those who are not likely to benefit from any surgical procedure, and those for whom the surgery would be equivocal. For the first group, the method could be subsequently used to compare the appropriateness of different procedures. This 2-step appropriateness classification could be conducted for a comprehensive set of patient scenarios covering most people presenting with pancreatic cancer. The scenarios could be designed to account for important factors used in devising a pancreatic cancer treatment plan, such as diagnostic study results, tumor features, presence of comorbidities, and patient preferences.

Another potential oncology topic might be colorectal cancer with hepatic metastases. The appropriateness method could be used to delineate which patients would benefit from surgical resection versus systemic chemotherapy. For those for whom surgery is appropriate, the method could be used to determine which patients would benefit from a simultaneous resection and which should undergo a staged resection. For breast cancer, the appropriateness method could be used to compare both the timing of surgery (ie, before or after neoadjuvant therapy) and the choice of surgical procedure (ie, lumpectomy with radiation therapy vs mastectomy). For women undergoing mastectomy, the method could be further used to determine the appropriateness of immediate versus delayed reconstruction, taking into account factors such as local advancement of the tumor.

Other procedures in surgical oncology would also benefit from application of the appropriateness method. In this article, we describe the method in greater detail and summarize 2 studies that used it to evaluate treatment options for patients with cancer. We conclude by suggesting how the results of the appropriateness method can be applied in real-world clinical settings.

THE APPROPRIATENESS METHOD

Randomized controlled trials are considered the gold standard for determining the safety and effectiveness of a procedure; however, the generalizability of trial results to a broad population is often limited by the reality that trials usually enroll a narrow spectrum of patients. In addition, relying on trials to determine the best treatment for a wide range of clinical scenarios would be impractical. The appropriateness method thus supplements evidence from clinical trials with expert opinion to better inform clinicians and patients regarding treatment options. The method was originally developed as a means of systematically defining which patients should and should not undergo surgery for a specific condition. It has subsequently also been used to compare the appropriateness of different procedures for the same indication; for example, percutaneous coronary intervention versus CABG for coronary artery disease.[1,2]

The appropriateness method starts with an extensive review of the literature on the risks and benefits of a procedure. A comprehensive and mutually exclusive set of clinical scenarios or indications for the procedure is then compiled, complete with specific definitions for any potentially ambiguous terms. Because the list needs to be inclusive, it typically includes many hundreds of clinical indications. Multidisciplinary panelists then weigh the relative risks and benefits of the procedure for each indication and assign ratings based on the best available evidence and his/her own clinical judgment. Rating usually occurs in 2 rounds, with the second round occurring after an in-person discussion of the first round results. Of note, the appropriateness method does not force panelists to come to a consensus on the appropriateness of an indication and each panelist rates each indication anonymously.

Indications are classified as "appropriate" (the expected benefits of the procedure outweigh the expected harms), "equivocal" (the expected benefits and harms are roughly equal or there is disagreement among the panelists), or "inappropriate" (the expected harms outweigh the expected benefits). Appropriate indications are sometimes further classified as "necessary" by the panel, usually in a third round. An indication is considered "necessary" if it would be improper care to not offer the procedure, there is a reasonable chance the procedure will benefit the patient, and the magnitude of the benefit is not small.[2] **Table 1** shows examples of indications with each of these classifications.

A substantial amount of research has been performed regarding the reliability and validity of the appropriateness method. Studies of test-retest reliability of the same panelists resulted in a correlation coefficient greater than 0.9.[10] Independent panels with the same composition of panelist disciplines generate results that are about as reproducible as some common diagnostic tests (kappa ~0.5–0.7).[5] The results of the appropriateness method are known to be sensitive to panel composition: physicians who perform the procedure are more enthusiastic about its appropriateness than those who do not perform the procedure.[11] Finally, predictive validity has been demonstrated for coronary revascularization, with patients who undergo treatment concordant with appropriateness classification having better outcomes than patients who undergo discordant care. For example, a prospective study on the appropriate use of coronary revascularization found that underuse was significantly associated with the adverse clinical outcomes of nonfatal myocardial infarction and mortality.[12]

SURGICAL APPROPRIATENESS CRITERIA FOR PATIENTS WITH CANCER

A number of studies have developed quality indicators for cancer care using a variation of the appropriateness method; however, relatively few have focused on developing appropriateness criteria (ie, balance of risks and benefits associated with surgical

Table 1
Examples of indications classified as "appropriate," "equivocal," or "inappropriate" for a specific procedure by a multidisciplinary panel using the appropriateness method

Procedure	Indication	Classification
Sentinel lymph node biopsy in melanoma[a]	Patient has a 1.1–4.0 mm lesion on the trunk without ulceration and classified Clark level 2 or 3.	Appropriate
	Patient has a 0.76–1.0 mm lesion on the extremity without ulceration and classified Clark level 2 or 3.	Equivocal
	Patient has a ≤0.75 mm lesion on the head without ulceration and classified as Clark level 2 or 3.	Inappropriate
Cytoreductive nephrectomy for metastatic renal cell cancer[b]	Patient with primary tumor in situ who has not received prior immunotherapy and has: • Limited metastatic burden, and • Targeted therapy planned, and • GOOD surgical risk, and • Symptoms related to primary tumor.	Appropriate
	Patient with primary tumor in situ who has not received prior immunotherapy and has: • Limited metastatic burden, and • Targeted therapy planned, and • GOOD surgical risk, and • NO symptoms related to primary tumor.	Equivocal
	Patient with primary tumor in situ who has not received prior immunotherapy and has: • Limited metastatic burden, and • Targeted therapy planned, and • POOR surgical risk, and • NO symptoms related to primary tumor.	Inappropriate

[a] The appropriateness study on sentinel lymph node biopsy in melanoma rated 48 indications that were constructed based on permutations of the following clinical factors: location of the lesion, Breslow depth, Clark level, and presence of ulceration.[13]

[b] The appropriateness study on cytoreductive nephrectomy for metastatic renal cell cancer rated 24 indications that were based on permutations of the following clinical factors: surgical risk, symptoms related to the primary tumor, metastatic burden, and prior immunotherapy versus plan for immunotherapy versus plan for targeted therapy.[14]

intervention for specific indications). We summarize 2 studies that used the appropriateness method for a surgical oncology topic.

The appropriateness method was used to develop criteria for sentinel lymph node biopsy and adjuvant high-dose interferon alfa-2b in melanoma. The study authors noted controversy surrounding the procedure and treatment because of a lack of definitive evidence in the literature. Their aim was to develop appropriateness criteria that could guide clinical decision making in practice. A multidisciplinary panel was convened comprising 4 dermatologists, 4 medical oncologists, and 5 surgical oncologists from geographically diverse areas and both community and academic settings. The panel rated 104 indications that were constructed based on the location of the lesion, Breslow depth, Clark level, presence of ulceration, lymph node involvement, and presence of micrometastases versus macrometastases. Of the indications for sentinel lymph node biopsy, 88% were rated appropriate and 6% inappropriate for the procedure. For interferon alfa-2b therapy, 89% of indications were rated appropriate and 9% inappropriate for this therapy. Examples of rated indications are shown in **Table 1**.[13]

The appropriateness method has also been used to evaluate treatment options for patients with metastatic renal cell cancer. A multidisciplinary panel composed of 2 urologists and 7 oncologists rated 108 indications for systemic therapy and 24 indications for cytoreductive nephrectomy. Indications were designed to represent clinical scenarios most likely to be seen in practice and included specifications of surgical risk, symptoms related to the primary tumor, previous or planned treatments, metastatic burden, and prognostic factors. Key terms, such as surgical risk, were explicitly defined. Of all the indications, 27% were rated appropriate and 47% were rated inappropriate. Examples of rated indications are shown in **Table 1**.[14]

Of note, the frequency of appropriate and inappropriate indications in these studies does not reflect the appropriateness of care for actual patients. When applied to specific patient populations, the appropriateness criteria may reveal higher or lower observed frequencies of appropriate care.

IMPLEMENTATION OF APPROPRIATENESS CRITERIA

Developing appropriateness criteria is only the first step toward improving patient selection for surgery. There are a number of ways in which the criteria can be implemented in both research and clinical settings. For some surgical procedures, appropriateness criteria have been applied to populations of actual patients to identify overuse and underuse. Overuse is generally defined as any instance in which a patient undergoes a procedure for an "inappropriate" indication, whereas underuse is defined as a patient with a "necessary" indication who does not receive the procedure. Studies on overuse in US populations report rates ranging from 9% to 53% for carotid endarterectomy[15,16] and 16% to 70% for hysterectomy.[6,17] Underuse has been studied in the US only for CABG, with reported rates ranging from 24% to 57%.[18,19]

Application of appropriateness criteria to actual patient populations can help determine if observed variation in the use of a surgical procedure is a result of overuse, underuse, or both. For patients with cancer, the likelihood of undergoing a surgical procedure can be quite different, even among neighboring regions with very similar populations. For example, in 2007, some regions performed as many as 4 times more inpatient mastectomies for cancer than other regions (0.42–1.69 per 1000 female Medicare enrollees, national average 1.00) and more than 6 times as many inpatient radical prostatectomies (0.55–3.67 per 1000 male Medicare enrollees, national average 1.59), even after adjusting for age and race.[20] The appropriateness method can be used to better understand why such variation occurs.

Geographic variation in use is probably not caused entirely by overuse in high-use regions, however. Researchers found only small differences in appropriate use of carotid endarterectomy, upper gastrointestinal endoscopy, and coronary angiography when appropriateness criteria were applied to patient populations in regions of high, average, and low use. For example, the percentage of carotid endarterectomies performed in the high-use and low-use regions that were found to be inappropriate (ie, overuse) was 30% and 29%, respectively. Because of such patterns, researchers suggest that geographic variation may result from combinations of overuse and underuse, along with other potential causes, such as differences in referral patterns and patient factors.[21]

The results of appropriateness studies also could be used to develop a comparative effectiveness research agenda by identifying gaps in knowledge. Procedures with a large number of equivocal indications highlight specific areas of uncertainty that could potentially be addressed by future experimental or observational trials.

Appropriateness criteria could be implemented in clinical settings, as well; not to replace a physician's clinical judgment, but rather to augment or guide decision making.[22] Some groups have developed computer algorithms based on the results of panel ratings, thus making appropriateness criteria more accessible and feasible for use in the clinical setting. With the rapid expansion of health information technology, such algorithms could be integrated into electronic medical records, streamlining appropriateness assessments for patients being considered for surgery. In this role, appropriateness criteria would serve as decision support for surgeons and referring physicians and could be considered as an electronic second opinion. Such clinical use of appropriateness criteria could be an effective way of reducing practice variation and improving the overall appropriateness of surgical care. This hypothesis is supported by a study that found that patient-specific appropriateness ratings were more effective than guidelines in changing the way that physicians treated angina.[23]

Appropriateness criteria could also be used to improve shared decision making between surgeons and patients by integrating personalized appropriateness assessments into the current informed consent process. Routinely supplying this information as a resource for patients is consistent with the current emphasis on providing patient-centered care. Indications classified as "equivocal" for a procedure could trigger a multidisciplinary effort to help patients decide whether to undergo surgery or proceed with other options.

Finally, administrators or health agencies could implement appropriateness criteria as a quality metric. As such, appropriateness criteria could be considered a process measure (ie, was appropriateness assessed and incorporated into the decision-making process or was the patient provided information on the appropriateness of surgical intervention) or as an outcome measure (ie, rates of overuse and underuse). An example of using appropriateness criteria as a quality metric is the Accreditation for Cardiovascular Excellence (ACE) program, which is a mandatory accrediting process proposed by the American College of Cardiology and the Society for Cardiovascular Angiography and Interventions in response to allegations of inappropriate use of percutaneous coronary intervention (PCI) in Maryland hospitals. Along with various process and outcome standards, a key component of the ACE accreditation is documentation of the indication for PCI and assessment of appropriateness using the current Appropriate Use Criteria for Coronary Artery Revascularization.[24,25]

SUMMARY

With the increasing focus on improving quality and promoting patient-centered care, ensuring that patients receive appropriate surgical procedures should be paramount. Current high-profile quality improvement efforts for the field of surgery, such as the Surgical Care Improvement Project, the American College of Surgeons (ACS) Commission on Cancer, and the ACS National Surgical Quality Improvement Program focus on improving processes and outcomes of care. Although these efforts are certainly critical for improving quality, they do not address whether patients are undergoing appropriate surgical procedures. A coordinated effort to produce appropriateness criteria for surgical oncology could potentially greatly improve the quality of surgical care for patients with cancer if these criteria are integrated into routine clinical practice. Some professional societies, such as the American College of Cardiology and the American College of Radiology, have already undertaken such programs. Surgical oncology could benefit from similar initiatives.

REFERENCES

1. Brook RH, Chassin MR, Fink A, et al. A method for the detailed assessment of the appropriateness of medical technologies. Int J Technol Assess Health Care 1986; 2(1):53–63.
2. Fitch K, Bernstein S, Aguilar M, et al. The RAND/UCLA appropriateness method user's manual 2001. No. MR-1269-DG-XII/RE:126. Santa Monica, CA: RAND Corp; 2001.
3. Park RE, Fink A, Brook RH, et al. Physician ratings of appropriate indications for six medical and surgical procedures. Am J Public Health 1986;76(7):766–72.
4. Burnand B, Vader JP, Froehlich F, et al. Reliability of panel-based guidelines for colonoscopy: an international comparison. Gastrointest Endosc 1998;47(2): 162–6.
5. Shekelle PG, Kahan JP, Bernstein SJ, et al. The reproducibility of a method to identify the overuse and underuse of medical procedures. N Engl J Med 1998; 338(26):1888–95.
6. Broder MS, Kanouse DE, Mittman BS, et al. The appropriateness of recommendations for hysterectomy. Obstet Gynecol 2000;95(2):199–205.
7. Yermilov I, McGory ML, Shekelle PW, et al. Appropriateness criteria for bariatric surgery: beyond the NIH guidelines. Obesity (Silver Spring) 2009;17(8):1521–7.
8. Kahan JP, Bernstein SJ, Leape LL, et al. Measuring the necessity of medical procedures. Med Care 1994;32(4):357–65.
9. Singh K, Lee BL, Wilson MR. A panel assessment of glaucoma management: modification of existing RAND-like methodology for consensus in ophthalmology. Part II: results and interpretation. Am J Ophthalmol 2008;145(3):575–81.
10. Merrick NJ, Fink A, Park RE, et al. Derivation of clinical indications for carotid endarterectomy by an expert panel. Am J Public Health 1987;77(2):187–90.
11. Kahan JP, Park RE, Leape LL, et al. Variations by specialty in physician ratings of the appropriateness and necessity of indications for procedures. Med Care 1996; 34(6):512–23.
12. Hemingway H, Crook AM, Feder G, et al. Underuse of coronary revascularization procedures in patients considered appropriate candidates for revascularization. N Engl J Med 2001;344(9):645–54.
13. Dubois RW, Swetter SM, Atkins M, et al. Developing indications for the use of sentinel lymph node biopsy and adjuvant high-dose interferon alfa-2b in melanoma. Arch Dermatol 2001;137(9):1217–24.
14. Halbert RJ, Figlin RA, Atkins MB, et al. Treatment of patients with metastatic renal cell cancer: a RAND Appropriateness Panel. Cancer 2006;107(10):2375–83.
15. Halm EA, Tuhrim S, Wang JJ, et al. Has evidence changed practice? Appropriateness of carotid endarterectomy after the clinical trials. Neurology 2007; 68(3):187–94.
16. Matchar DB, Oddone EZ, McCrory DC, et al. Influence of projected complication rates on estimated appropriate use rates for carotid endarterectomy. Appropriateness Project Investigators. Academic Medical Center Consortium. Health Serv Res 1997;32(3):325–42.
17. Bernstein SJ, McGlynn EA, Siu AL, et al. The appropriateness of hysterectomy. A comparison of care in seven health plans. Health Maintenance Organization Quality of Care Consortium. JAMA 1993;269(18):2398–402.
18. Epstein AM, Weissman JS, Schneider EC, et al. Race and gender disparities in rates of cardiac revascularization: do they reflect appropriate use of procedures or problems in quality of care? Med Care 2003;41(11):1240–55.

19. Conigliaro J, Whittle J, Good CB, et al. Understanding racial variation in the use of coronary revascularization procedures: the role of clinical factors. Arch Intern Med 2000;160(9):1329–35.
20. The Dartmouth Atlas of Health Care. Understanding of the efficiency and effectiveness of the health care system. Available at: http://www.dartmouthatlas.org/. Accessed August 29, 2011.
21. Chassin MR, Kosecoff J, Park RE, et al. Does inappropriate use explain geographic variations in the use of health care services? A study of three procedures. JAMA 1987;258(18):2533–7.
22. Brook RH. Assessing the appropriateness of care—its time has come. JAMA 2009;302(9):997–8.
23. Junghans C, Feder G, Timmis AD, et al. Effect of patient-specific ratings vs conventional guidelines on investigation decisions in angina: Appropriateness of Referral and Investigation in Angina (ARIA) Trial. Arch Intern Med 2007; 167(2):195–202.
24. Brindis R, Goldberg SD, Turco MA, et al. President's page: quality and appropriateness of care: the response to allegations and actions needed by the cardiovascular professional. J Am Coll Cardiol 2011;57(1):111–3.
25. ACE Standards for Catheterization Laboratory Accreditation: Accreditation for Cardiovascular Excellence; 2011. Available at: http://www.cvexcel.org/Default.aspx. Accessed March 14, 2012.

Collaboration with the Community Cancer Center
Benefit for All

Nicholas J. Petrelli, MD[a],*, Patrick Grusenmeyer, ScD[b]

KEYWORDS

- Community • Cancer • Translational • Trials • Cancer control • Genetic counseling
- Multidisciplinary centers • Translational research

KEY POINTS

- Successful community centers should have (1) program development with a core comprising high-quality well-trained professionals, (2) resources, (3) collaboration with institutions of higher learning, and (4) collaboration with community organizations.
- The National Cancer Institute Community Cancer Centers Program involves 7 pillars of care and research, including disparities, clinical trials, patient advocacy, biospecimen collection and preparation, and survivorship programs.
- Establishing genetic counseling and gene-testing programs is important to lower cancer incidence and mortality in any state. This effort needs to involve primary care physicians who refer patients to genetic counselors for evaluation and possible gene testing.
- The key to a successful disease site multidisciplinary center is a care coordinator or nurse navigator to coordinate scheduling and guide the patient through the complex maze of cancer care and follow-up. The nurse navigator is the key communicator to the patients and their families.
- The Center for Translational Cancer Research (CTCR) is a formal alliance between the University of Delaware, the Helen F. Graham Cancer Center, the Nemours Research Foundation/Alfred I. duPont Hospital for Children, and the Delaware Biotechnology Institute at the University of Delaware. The CTCR has created a center without walls to support clinical and basic science efforts within the state.

This project has been funded in whole or in part with federal funds from the National Cancer Institute, National Institutes of Health, under the contract number HHSN261200800001E. The content of this publication does not necessarily reflect the views or policies of the Department of Health and Human Services, nor does mention of trade names, commercial products, or organizations imply endorsement by the US Government.
The authors have nothing to disclose.
[a] Helen F. Graham Cancer Center, 4701 Ogletown-Stanton Road, Suite 1233, Newark, DE 19713, USA; [b] Cancer and Imaging Services, Helen F. Graham Cancer Center, Christiana Care Health System, 4701 Ogletown-Stanton Road, Newark, DE 19713, USA
* Corresponding author. Helen F. Graham Cancer Center, Christiana Care Health System, 4701 Ogletown-Stanton Road, Newark, DE 19713.
E-mail address: npetrelli@christianacare.org

1055-3207/12/$ – see front matter © 2012 Elsevier Inc. All rights reserved.

Building a quality community cancer center takes a significant amount of work, and a vision that is both practical and cutting edge. For a community cancer center to be successful, several components are required:

1. Program development must have access to a core of high-quality well-trained professionals.
2. Resources must be available.
3. Collaboration with institutions of higher learning is critical.
4. Collaboration with community cancer organizations is critical.

Equipping a community cancer center to the level of an academic center requires the collaboration of several institutions. The Helen F. Graham Cancer Center (HFGCC) at Christiana Care is fortunate to have strong collaborative efforts and research agreements with the University of Delaware and the Kimmel Cancer Center at Thomas Jefferson University. The center has also been fortunate to have an outstanding relationship with community cancer organizations, such as the American Cancer Society, the Leukemia and Lymphoma Society, the Delaware Breast Cancer Coalition, and the Wellness Community.[1] Collaboration through a strong state cancer control program is another important component for a successful community cancer center. Delaware has one of the best state cancer control programs in the United States. In 2001 the Delaware Cancer Consortium was formed, which, in 2002, launched its first statewide program to screen all Delawareans older than 50 years with colonoscopy. These results are further discussed in this article.

In May 2007, the HFGCC became 1 of the 16 members of the original National Cancer Institute Community Cancer Centers Program (NCCCP) to allow access to the cancer Biomedical Informatics Grid (caBIG) of the National Cancer Institute (NCI) and The Cancer Genome Atlas project; this is also discussed in this article.

PARTICIPATION IN THE NCCCP

The NCCCP involves 7 pillars of care and research:

1. Disparities
2. Clinical trials, especially increasing minority accrual to clinical trials
3. Patient advocacy
4. Biospecimen collection and preparation
5. Survivorship programs
6. Quality of care, including the multidisciplinary approach to cancer care
7. Information technology with implementation of electronic health record.

The NCCCP involves a network of 16 original institutions, which increased to a total of 30 in the spring of 2010. Disparities overtake all of the 7 pillars of the NCCCP. This program was the concept of John Niederhuber, MD, former Director of the NCI. The program came into existence because Dr Niederhuber realized that 85% of patients with cancer in the United States are diagnosed at community hospitals with the remaining 15% diagnosed at the NCI-designated cancer centers, which are mainly located in urban areas. It is also known that many patients are not treated at the NCI-designated cancer centers because of economic reasons, distance from home, or personal reasons. The mission of the NCCCP is to enhance cancer care at community hospitals and also to create a platform to support basic, clinical, and population-based research. As of now, the 30 NCCCP sites located in 22 states are developing and evaluating programs to enhance community-based cancer care and create a community cancer center network to support research. This network also supports research in collaboration with the NCI-designated Cancer Centers Program, The Cancer Genome Atlas project, the American Society of Clinical Oncology, and the American College of Surgeons Commission on Cancer. In the area of enhanced community-based cancer care, the institutions in this network are reducing disparities in cancer health care across the cancer continuum, at the same time improving quality of cancer care and expanding survivorship and palliative care programs. In the area of cancer research initiatives, the NCCCP institutions support the investigation of new drugs through clinical trials, increasing the quality of biospecimen collection procedures for research through a standardized base approach and expanding information technology capabilities through electronic medical records and, as mentioned earlier, the NCI's caBIG. Examples of some of these projects are as follows:

1. To meet the NCI's need for standardized data, the NCCCP hospitals have united in their approach to collecting race and ethnicity data. The NCCCP sites are standardizing race and ethnicity data collection using the US Office of Management and Budget guidelines and categories.
2. The NCCCP sites, through their staff, have embraced the need for improved cultural awareness of specific populations to make progress toward reducing health care disparities. The sites have worked with individuals in the field and patient advocates to develop webinars exploring the health histories and beliefs of African Americans and Native Americans.
3. The NCCCP sites, along with the American College of Surgeons Commission on Cancer, are testing the Rapid Quality Reporting System of the Commission. This system provides real-time surveillance and feedback to centers on the status of patients whose cancer care falls within the National Comprehensive Cancer Network (NCCN) guidelines.
4. The NCCCP sites are working with their community-based private practice oncologists in participating in the American Society of Clinical Oncology's Quality Oncology Practice Initiative. This initiative involves monitoring physician adherence to evidence-based guidelines for treatment and surveillance.

These are but a few examples of the projects that the NCCCP is involved in. The projects have been successful because of the participation of private practice oncologists of all cancer disciplines. The NCCCP is a model network wherein institutions share best practices and are involved in continued communication across all 7 pillars to improve patient care and research.

STATE CANCER CONTROL PROGRAM

The state of Delaware reports approximately 4600 new cancer cases on an annual basis. In 2010 the overall population of Delaware was 876,653. The most common cancers in the state are those that are reflected nationally: lung, breast, prostate, and colorectal cancers. A substantial number of melanomas are diagnosed each year because of the existence of beaches in the southern part of the state and subsequent unprotected sun exposure. In the past, Delaware was ranked number 1 in the United States for both cancer incidence and mortality. In view of the success of many screening, treatment, and genetic counseling/gene-testing programs, Delaware's mortality rate is dropping twice as fast as the national rate. A major impact has been the Clean Indoor Air Act passed in November 2002, which, along with the statewide colorectal screening program, constitutes the 2 main reasons for the improvement of cancer statistics in the state of Delaware. The Delaware Cancer Treatment Program has been contributing to this success. Funds from the tobacco settlement have been used to establish the Delaware Cancer Treatment Program. An uninsured family of 4 in the state of Delaware earning up to $120,000 per year can receive 2 years of cancer treatment. The individual simply has to be a resident of the state. In addition, in 2007 an education program for the human papillomavirus vaccine was started, which continues to this day and which in the future will certainly have a dramatic impact on cervical cancer incidence across the country.

Before 2002, there was not a single full-time adult genetic counselor in the state. At present, there are 4 full-time adult genetic counselors at the HFGCC who serve the state of Delaware. A high-risk family cancer registry named after the former governor of the state, Ruth Ann Minner, has been established. This registry has more than 100,000 individuals and 2000 families. The bar graph in **Fig. 1** demonstrates the number of patients offered genetic testing and the actual number of patients who underwent testing from 2002 to 2011; the dramatic increase in both is self-explanatory. This increase has taken a tremendous educational effort on the part of the genetic counselors with both physicians and the public.

In 2008, Delaware was ranked fifth for breast cancer screening in the United States. In the following year the state was ranked first for colorectal cancer screening. In 2010, Delaware's adult smoking rate was 17.8%, which is the lowest in the state's history and below the national rate of 19%. Results of the Statewide Colorectal Screening Program have demonstrated that in 2008, Delaware's colorectal cancer screening rate for Caucasians was 17% higher than the national rate. For African Americans, the rate in Delaware was 25% higher than the national rate. Just as importantly, in 2008 the disparity between African Americans and Caucasians for colorectal screening endoscopies was eliminated.

GENETIC COUNSELING AND GENE TESTING: A COLLABORATIVE EFFORT

The success of any community cancer program takes collaborative efforts on the part of both individuals and organizations. On a weekly basis, the genetic counselors at the HFGCC visit the Tunnell Cancer Center at the Beebe Medical Center in Sussex County, which is located in the southern part of the state. The Tunnell Cancer Center

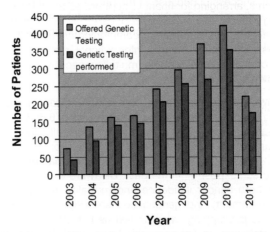

Fig. 1. Genetic testing per year. The number of individuals who were offered genetic testing through the Ruth Ann Minner High Risk Family Cancer Registry and the number of individuals who actually underwent gene testing after genetic counseling at the HFGCC from 2001 to May 2011.

is under the direction of James Spellman, MD, a surgical oncologist by training who is also the American College of Surgeons Commission on Cancer State Liaison for Delaware. Along with medical and radiation oncologists at the Tunnell Cancer Center, for the past 8 years a collaborative effort has existed not only with the genetic counseling program but also with the NCI Community Clinical Oncology Program (CCOP). The Beebe Medical Center is a satellite of the HFGCC/Christiana Care CCOP. Clinical trials and collaborations and genetic counseling/gene testing are 2 successful programs between both institutions. The presence of genetic counselors at the Tunnell Cancer Center avoids the need for patients in Sussex County to travel to the northern part of the state to see genetic counselors for evaluation. After evaluation, if patients are recommended that they undergo prophylactic surgery, these patients are referred back to the Tunnell Cancer Center for surgery. The genetic counseling program has also been successful in the middle part of the state, Kent County. This collaborative effort involves primary care physicians who refer patients to the genetic counselors for evaluation and possible gene testing. The program results of individuals with genetic alterations have resulted in 90% to 95% of family members having an impact on their health care management. There is no question that the recommendations of prophylactic surgery, chemoprevention, and increased surveillance have had a positive impact on cancer statistics in the state of Delaware.

THE NCI CCOP

The Christiana Care/HFGCC research program is staffed by 27.5 full-time equivalents. This includes a director, 5 nurse coordinators, 15.5 research nurses, 2 clinical research associates, and 4 administrative assistants. This team supports 6 physician practices and 27 physicians (medical oncologists/hematologists/radiation and surgical oncologists). Coverage is also provided to the HFGCC multidisciplinary disease site centers (MDCs; discussed in detail later in this article). The program also includes a dedicated investigational oncology pharmacy service. Since 1987, when the NCI CCOP was initially funded, Christiana Care has steadily improved in meeting its accrual requirements to clinical trials.

The CCOP is well represented within the National Cooperative Study Groups. Representation includes appointments with 25 separate cooperative group committees. The CCOP is frequently recognized as being among the top accruing institutions for the Radiation Therapy Oncology Group (RTOG) and the Cancer and Leukemia Group B (CALGB). In 2004, the American Society of Clinical Oncology recognized the program with a Clinical Trials Participation Award for accrual to RTOG trials. The CCOP was profiled in the July 2006 NCI Cancer Bulletin. In 2010, the CALGB recognized the CCOP as the highest accruer to NCI clinical trials among all CALGB CCOPs. Over the past 20 years, the HFGCC/Christiana Care CCOP has enrolled more than 5000 participants to the NCI-approved Cooperative Group clinical trials. During the calendar year 2009, Christiana Care diagnosed a total of 3094 analytic cancer cases; of those, 719 patients or 23.1% of individuals participated in a clinical trial, ranking Christiana Care as one of the highest accruing institutions in the United States. In 2010, the accrual rate was 22%. An average of 125 NCI active clinical trials is available at any given time, giving access to protocols for all disease sites. The success of the accrual rate can be attributed to several factors. First, the established MDCs are staffed by clinical research nurses as part of the multidisciplinary team. The research nurses are well aware of the details of the clinical trials. Second, clinical research nurses are housed in the physicians' private office only if they meet the performance expectations of the cancer program. Third, there is a monthly CCOP newsletter that is shared with satellites and a monthly CCOP meeting with trial review so that trials not accruing during a certain period of time are brought to the attention of the CCOP group and are emphasized at the tumor conferences. Another contributing factor to the high accrual rate is the annual CCOP symposium, where awards are given to the high-accruing physicians. These awards are given to surgeons who receive accrual credit when they refer a patient to a medical or radiation oncologist and that patient participates in a clinical trial.

A table demonstrating accrual in the areas of treatment, cancer control, prevention, and pharmaceutical and translational research trials are shared on a monthly basis with all physicians. Thereby, individual physicians know where they stand with their colleagues in terms of accrual.

In January 2008, a new program was started to help increase the accrual rate to NCI clinical trials. The program involves clinical trial investigators earning their status as an investigator.[2] Several criteria are required for physicians to maintain their status as clinical trials investigator. These include:

1. A minimum of 4 patients accrued per calendar year to NCI clinical trials
2. Attendance in one NCI Cooperative Group or CCOP research base meeting every year
3. Medical records that must undergo an audit in preparation for NCI Cooperative Group audits.

Failure to meet these criteria means a loss of clinical trials investigator status. Physicians can be reinstated, but they must wait for 1 year, attend an NCI Cooperative Group meeting, and then pay a fee of $500. Since 2008, this program has been very successful as it continues to reach the goal of a 30% accrual rate to NCI clinical trials by 2014.

ESTABLISHING MDCs

The MDCs at the HFGCC have been very successful. This project required the buy-in of private practice physicians with the vision that better and more efficient care would be achieved when patients and their family members are seen in a group setting in which the 3 major disciplines of surgery, medical oncology, and radiation oncology along with support services occurred. The key to a successful MDC is a care coordinator or nurse navigator whose duty is to coordinate scheduling and guide the patient through the complex maze of cancer care and follow-up. The nurse navigator is the key communicator to the patient and his or her family. There should also be coordinated support care services, such as pastoral care, social service, nutrition, and pain and palliative care. The medical director and vice president of the cancer program must work together with legal counsel to develop a model that can optimize professional facility fee billing, especially in community cancer centers where most physicians are in private practice.

Multidisciplinary centers differ from tumor conferences in several ways. The major difference is that at an MDC, the patient together with friends and/or family are physically present to discuss recommendations with the multidisciplinary care team. In general, this is not the case at tumor conferences. In the environment of the multidisciplinary center, the patient's treatment plan is also established within a shorter time frame because face-to-face discussions occur with the 3 major disciplines of surgery, radiation, and medical/hematologic oncology along with any of the necessary support services. This also results in fewer biased decisions. This is classically demonstrated in a genitourinary multidisciplinary center where the radiation oncologist and urologic surgeon must have a face-to-face discussion on the best treatment approach for a patient with the diagnosis of prostate cancer. The MDCs are also important in helping to increase accrual to clinical trials because the clinical research nurse is an important member of the multidisciplinary team.

There are several key elements to starting an MDC or clinic (**Box 1**). Also important is a physician who can direct the center members and keep them on track so that the process runs smoothly and efficiently. A financial expert is needed to design and review the billing plan with hospital and legal counsel. A committee to design and review performance criteria and outcomes in patients needs to be formed so that physicians maintain high-quality cancer care. The required performance expectations at the HFGCC include a 66% annual attendance at tumor conferences, maintaining a publication record or presentations at regional/national oncology conferences, and participation in professional cancer organizations both nationally and locally, among others.

Private practice physicians who participate in the MDCs do their own billing. This process needs to be explained before the MDC team sees patients. An example would be a patient who presents to the MDC with esophageal cancer. If the MDC team decides that surgery would be the upfront treatment, the surgeon would likely bill the level 5 charge, and the medical oncologist and radiation oncologist would be the 2 consultants explaining to the patient the possible need for chemoradiation postoperatively; however, because each physician does his or her billing independently, the charge is determined based on the services rendered and documented. Performance improvements of the multidisciplinary team are an important factor in providing high-quality cancer care. An interesting project by the original 16 NCCCP sites was started in the fall of 2010. The study examines the association between the intensity of individual multidisciplinary center models and the short-term patient outcomes at the NCCCP sites. The variations across the 16 NCCCP pilot sites in their baseline multidisciplinary cancer care measures, practices, and outcomes, over time, are studied. The outcomes to be examined in this project include (1) time from initial pathology diagnosis to commencement of therapy, (2) use of treatment modalities recommended by the NCCN guidelines, and (3) patient satisfaction. Quantitative measures are drawn from the NCCCP data on multidisciplinary centers, and linked to patient data that are collected and submitted to the American College of Surgeons Commission on Cancer for inclusion in the National Cancer Data Base through each site's tumor registry. At the patient level, sampling focuses on patients with solid tumors who are potential candidates for multimodality therapy during the early part of their treatment. This sampling includes patients who are newly diagnosed with stage III lung cancer and stage II and III colorectal cancers. Successful completion of this project is likely to have a positive impact on the delivery of cancer care in the community setting, with similar implications possible in the academic setting. It is hoped that through the use of data from the

---

Box 1
Key elements in the multidisciplinary process

- Assign a nurse navigator to coordinate scheduling and guide the patient through the complex maze of cancer care.

- Centralize registration for one point of entry for the patient and use of information technology to communicate it systemwide.

- Coordinate supportive care services.

- Develop a model that can optimize professional and facility fee billing.

- Ensure that all elements support an efficiently run system.

NCCCP sites, this study will generate additional knowledge about whether multidisciplinary cancer care improves the timeliness of treatment and patient satisfaction and ultimately leads to improved outcomes in patients.

The American College of Surgeons Commission on Cancer realizes that cancer conferences play an integral part in improving the care of patients with cancer. The HFGCC has been successful in establishing a statewide community cancer center videoconferencing program, reported in detail by Dickson-Witmer and colleagues.[3] In addition to the multidisciplinary centers at the HFGCC, the program also holds disease-site tumor conferences, at which discussions are held based on the NCCN or the American Society of Clinical Oncology guidelines for treatment and surveillance. For the last 3 years, compliance with guidelines has ranged between 85% and 95%.

THE CENTER FOR TRANSLATIONAL CANCER RESEARCH

February 1, 2006, marked the creation of the Center for Translational Cancer Research (CTCR) in the state of Delaware.[4] The CTCR is a formal alliance between the University of Delaware, the HFGCC, the Nemours/Alfred I. duPont Hospital for Children, and the Delaware Biotechnology Institute (DBI) at the University of Delaware. The CTCR has created a center without walls to support clinical and basic science efforts in translational cancer research within the state. The laboratory and offices of the Cancer Biomarkers and Genetics Program of the CTCR are located on the fourth floor of the HFGCC pavilion expansion, which was completed in June 2009. The CTCR in the HFGCC contains 6000 square feet of laboratory space. This project has led to matching HFGCC clinicians with scientists to foster better cancer care in the state. These teams consist of clinicians, scientists, genetic counselors, engineers, information technologists, and support staff. Some examples of these collaborative efforts are:

1. The discovery of a stem cell marker that makes it possible to track stem cell overpopulation during colon cancer development and the role of microRNAs in colon cancer development
2. Interaction of bone marrow stromal cells in the microenvironment with cancer cells that metastasize to the bone from prostate cancer
3. Development of targeted drugs for renal clear cell carcinoma
4. Tissue engineering replacement for head and neck cancers, such as artificial salivary glands to replace glands damaged by radiation therapy.[4]

The genetic aspect of the CTCR uses information from the previously described Ruth Ann Minner High Risk Family Cancer Registry. In this registry, often there are individuals from families with a strong history of cancer in each generation who test negative for known gene mutations. These individuals provide a means of discovering new cancer genes. One exciting new class of cancer genes is the microRNAs, which are inactive tumor suppressors and hence allow cancer to develop. The aim of the research program is to tap into the scientific expertise at the University of Delaware/DBI and Nemours/Alfred I. duPont Hospital for Children for the discovery of these new genes and their mutations, which can serve in population screening at the HFGCC. The resources to acquire the instruments needed to support all these projects have been obtained by grant funding whenever possible, but also through philanthropy.

The CTCR represents a model whereby community-based cancer centers can expand their impact on the communities they serve. With the partnering of interested basic science centers, stimulating exchange that strengthens all institutions and investigators involved can occur. The science that emerges is more attuned to issues

---

Box 2
DHSA: March 2009

- Collaborations in education, research and development, personnel
- Initial focus on cancer and cardiovascular research
- Efforts in rehabilitation and neuroscience
- Future development of the Delaware Center for Cancer Biology

---

of patient care, which include diagnosis, treatment, and prognosis. Basic science also benefits from a better understanding of the state of the art and disease management, outcomes, and presentation. Graduate and undergraduate students at the university level benefit from clinical exposure, which would be impossible without the formalized interactions established in the CTCR. On the other hand, surgical and medical residents are beginning to benefit from research years that immerse them in the university environment and bench science.

In the spring of 2009, the Delaware Health Sciences Alliance (DHSA) was formed between the Thomas Jefferson University, the University of Delaware, the Alfred I. duPont Children's Hospital, and the Christiana Care Health System. The collaborative effort of these 4 institutions will lead to the establishment of a medical school in Delaware, which will be an extension of the Jefferson Medical College. The success of the CTCR will lead to the establishment of the Delaware Center for Cancer Biology. The Delaware Center for Cancer Biology plans to house cancer genetics, immunology, biology, and drug development. The 4 areas of focus for the DHSA are cancer, cardiovascular research, rehabilitation, and neuroscience (**Box 2**).

In conclusion, developing successful programs in a community cancer center involves the collaborative efforts of employed and private practice physicians, hospital and cancer center administrations, significant resources, and support personnel, coupled with a vision that will lead to improved patient outcomes and cancer care.

REFERENCES

1. Petrelli N. A community cancer center: getting to the next level. J Am Coll Surg 2010;210(3):261–70.
2. Petrelli N, Grubbs S, Price K. Clinical trial investigator status: you need to earn it. J Clin Oncol 2008;26:2440–1.
3. Dickson-Witmer D, Petrelli N, Witmer D, et al. A statewide community cancer center videoconferencing program. Ann Surg Oncol 2008;15:3058–64.
4. Sikes R, Duncan R, Lee K, et al. The Center for Translational Cancer Research: a collaborative effort between the Helen F. Graham Cancer Center at Christiana Care, the University of Delaware and Nemours Biomedical Research. Oncol Issues 2011;22–5.

Value-Based Health Care
A Surgical Oncologist's Perspective

Janice N. Cormier, MD, MPH*, Kate D. Cromwell, MS,
Raphael E. Pollock, MD

KEYWORDS

- Value-based health care • Medical practice units • Cost-effectiveness • Patient cost

KEY POINTS

- Value-based health care proposes a model that evaluates health care based on 6 elements: safety, effectiveness, patient centeredness, timeliness, efficiency, and equity.
- The primary goal of value-based health care is to achieve an optimal health outcome with consideration of dollars spent for care.
- An integrated practice unit of care allows coordination of care for patients across medical disciplines, which expedites treatment and eliminates duplication of services.
- Successful programs for value-based health care have been implemented for organ transplantation, coronary and dialysis care, and in vitro fertilization.

The quality of health care is difficult to define and even more challenging to measure. Practicing clinicians know that the quality of care a patient receives goes beyond issues of survival because treatment decisions affect many aspects of life.[1] Traditional components of health care quality have been broadly delineated as structure, process, and outcome measures.[2,3] Structure refers to institutional characteristics and procedural volumes. Process refers to the elements of care delivered and has most commonly been evaluated in terms of compliance with evidence-based care guidelines. Outcomes have been considered the most important and easily measured quality metric; these are most commonly represented as mortality and morbidity.

One of the many challenges in quality research has been the translation of each of these quality components into measureable indicators so as to monitor and improve the quality of care at the population level.[4,5] With respect to structure, surgical volumes have been the most extensively studied.[6–8] However, the strength of the relationship between structure and outcomes varies widely. Process measures are the most widely used quality-measurement metrics. In theory, process measures should

Financial disclosures and/or conflicts of interest: The authors have nothing to disclose.
Department of Surgical Oncology, Unit 444, The University of Texas MD Anderson Cancer Center, 1400 Holcombe Boulevard, Houston, TX 77030-4009, USA
* Corresponding author.
E-mail address: jcormier@mdanderson.org

doi:10.1016/j.soc.2012.03.001
1055-3207/12/$ – see front matter © 2012 Elsevier Inc. All rights reserved.
surgonc.theclinics.com

correlate with outcomes of care,[9] but such associations have been difficult to show. In addition, although process measures may be useful metrics for institutions, they are not a substitute for outcomes, which are considered the only true measures of quality in health care. For example, even with highly selected process indicators or treatment guidelines targeted for compliance, there may be legitimate reasons for an individual patient to not receive guideline-based care (eg, clinician propensity, practice barriers, medical contraindications, or patient preferences).[10,11] In addition, using adherence rates as a process measure is problematic because it can unintentionally promote the overuse of medical services.[12] Traditional outcome indicators include morbidity, which assesses the unintended consequences of treatment in a measureable way, and survival and recurrence, which indicate whether a treatment is achieving its intended goal. However, consensus definitions for disease-specific outcomes do not exist and the comprehensive systematic measurement of outcomes is rare.[13]

According to Michael E. Porter,[14] MBA, PhD, of the Harvard Business School, the Institute of Medicine's lack of clarity in defining the proposed 6 elements of quality health care (safety, effectiveness, patient centeredness, timeliness, efficiency, and equity[15]) has slowed progress in improving the performance of the health care system. To enhance the performance and accountability of the health care system, stakeholders must therefore abandon these individual quality-defining elements, which often represent conflicting goals, and concentrate on value as a single focus for health care delivery.[16] Porter[14] argues that the inability to measure value in health care has been the most serious failure in the medical community to date and has significantly impeded health care reform.[15]

VALUE-BASED HEALTH CARE

In contrast with more traditional measures of health care quality, the primary goal of value-based health care is to achieve good health outcomes for patients with consideration of dollars spent.[17] Value-based health care promotes a patient-centered program in which outcomes are evaluated by relevant patient outcomes rather than individual processes that contribute to outcomes. Another unique feature of value-based health care is that each medical condition has its own outcome measures that are precisely defined and assessed longitudinally. Along with disease-specific outcomes, total costs over time are considered to account for ongoing interventions and treatment-associated illnesses.[18] The premise for value-based health care is that, if value provides overall improvement in health care systems, then all stakeholders (including patients, payers, and providers) benefit and economic sustainability is maintained.[14,16]

One of the challenges in improving performance in health care has been in defining value, which, simply stated, is the patient health outcomes achieved plus the efficiency of the delivery of services as accounted for by costs.[14] In this system, outcomes include the "results of care in terms of patients' health over time"[13] with consideration of complications of care, timeliness of care, and patient satisfaction. The full cycle of care in value-based health care includes diagnostic evaluation, acute care, related early and late complications, rehabilitation, and reoccurrences. Unlike current mechanisms of evaluation, value-based health care is measured over time at disease-specific intervals.[13,19] These definitions of care and health are in contrast with those used in the current health care system, in which acute events are most often isolated from the care cycle and processes of care, or the volume of services delivered is often emphasized.

OUTCOME HIERARCHY

Given that, for any medical condition, there is no single outcome that captures the results of care in terms of patient health, proponents of value-based health care argue that the current system assesses outcomes in a manner that is either too broad or too narrow.[19] For example, a patient with breast cancer who is diagnosed as tumor free would be considered to have a positive outcome in the narrow definition of breast cancer outcomes, but that patient may have ongoing symptoms associated with treatment (eg, posttreatment lymphedema) that result in a less favorable overall outcome. Similarly, assessment and reporting of hospital infection rates, mortality, medication errors, or surgical complications are outcomes that are too broad to provide evaluation of a provider's care in a way that is meaningful for an individual patient, and they may also miss relevant treatment-associated complications and long-term sequelae.[13]

To address these limitations of the current system, 4 principles have been defined in the value-based health care model to determine relevant multidimensional and disease-specific outcome measures: (1) relevant outcomes should be defined for individual medical conditions, (2) both short-term and long-term outcomes associated with these conditions should be considered within a care cycle that has a specified beginning and end, (3) outcome measures should include the full spectrum of contributing services and providers, and (4) outcome measures should adjust for individual risk factors and comorbidities.[13]

Porter[19] proposed a 3-tiered hierarchy to account for the spectrum of outcomes for any medical condition (**Fig. 1**). In this model, tier 1 represents patient health status achieved or retained, tier 2 the process of recovery, and tier 3 the sustainability of

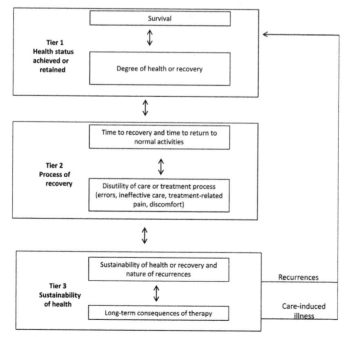

Fig. 1. The outcome measures hierarchy. (*Reprinted from* Porter ME. What is value in health care? N Engl J Med 2010;363(26):2479; with permission.)

health. The outcomes depend on a progression of results that, in turn, depend on the success at higher tiers.[16] Each tier consists of 2 dimensions that capture specific aspects of health.

Tier 1 is considered the most important of the three. The first dimension of tier 1 is patient survival, which is measured at condition-appropriate time intervals. The second dimension, degree of patient health or recovery, accounts for the full set of outcomes that are of significance to a patient and are related to the processes of recovery. Recovery is measured by the degree to which patients are able to return to their normal activities of daily living (ie, functional status) once condition-specific steady state has been achieved after treatment. For many cancers, recovery measures include functional outcomes, cosmetic results, and psychological state.[20]

Tier 2 of the outcome hierarchy accounts for the processes (rather than degree) of recovery. The first dimension of tier 2 assesses the patient's time to recovery and time to return to normal activities (ie, the best attainable level of function after diagnosis). This dimension is considered for each phase of care. Reducing the overall cycle time by reducing the time needed to complete various phases of care (eg, diagnosis, treatment planning, and initiation of treatment) is of major importance to patients.[13] The second dimension of tier 2 accounts for the disutility of care or treatment process, such as adverse effects, diagnostic errors, treatment-related pain, ineffective treatment, and condition-specific complications related to treatment.

Tier 3 accounts for the sustainability of health, which "measures the degree of health maintained as well as the extent and timing of related recurrences and consequences"[13] In this tier, the first dimension considers the recurrence of disease or long-term complications, whereas the second dimension captures new health conditions that occur as a consequence of treatment.

In this 3-tiered outcome model, improving 1 dimension benefits the others, and tradeoffs among outcome measures can be explicitly considered. For example, although there are limited treatment options for some metastatic cancers that do not influence survival (tier 1, first dimension) but may provide timely care, palliation of symptoms, and prolonged time to adverse consequences, thereby positively affecting tier 2 and tier 3 dimensions. An example of the hierarchical outcome model as applied for patients with locally advanced extremity soft tissue sarcoma is shown in **Fig. 2**.

Each medical condition is associated with a unique set of outcome dimensions. Defining these outcomes must consider their "importance to patient, variability, frequency, and practicality."[13] To successfully define outcomes, information should be sought from focus groups, families, and patient advisories. In this value-based system, validated instruments (eg, for functional outcomes or quality of life) can be used to assess individual dimensions and to compare health outcomes across providers. Another critical element to capturing quality data longitudinally is an information technology infrastructure that can facilitate the extraction of clinical data for measurement purposes.

In summary, accountability for the value of health care should be shared by all physicians. Extensive outcome hierarchies for specific medical conditions provide a comprehensive measurement system that may result in improvements in care at the level of health care providers. In addition, future public reporting of such outcomes could ultimately "accelerate innovation by motivating providers to improve relative to their peers."[16]

INTEGRATED PRACTICE UNITS

For the provision of value-based health care, Porter and colleagues[27,28] recently introduced the concept of integrated practice units (IPUs). These units are responsible for

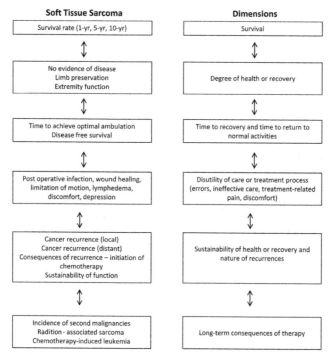

Fig. 2. Outcome hierarchy for locally advanced extremity soft tissue sarcoma.

the spectrum of providers and services for a particular medical condition and its complications.[16] IPUs include physicians and other staff who are disease-specific experts and can work together to offer the best and most efficient treatment and follow-up, thereby avoiding duplication of services and referrals.[21] In such a unit, there is greater emphasis on the relationship among physicians participating in an individual patient's care, which allows greater interconnectivity among the physicians and better coordination at each phase of treatment (spanning from disease prevention to post-treatment surveillance).[22] To be most efficient, an IPU should be physically located within the same facility.

The concept of IPUs was implemented in Finland beginning in the 1960s. As the Finnish system has become more fully established, infant mortality has decreased and life expectancy is increased while total medical expenditures in these areas have decreased.[21]

COSTS OF CARE

Improving efficiency has emerged as an urgent issue in health care. Current health care cost models are based on a fee-for-service reimbursement structure that collects costs from individual specialists, service areas, drugs, and supplies for individual events associated with a specific condition. One of the many challenges of this nonintegrated approach is that it provides incentives to maximize activity around the most profitable services and thus excess spending.

In contrast, with the value-based health care model, Porter and Teisberg[22] propose that costs should be measured over a patient's cycle of care and considered within the context of outcomes. Services should reflect all of the resources involved, including inpatient and outpatient treatment, drugs, devices, services, and rehabilitation, and should be based on a comparison of the benefits and all potential outcomes from the individual patient's perspective.[23] In addition to coordinating health care services and their associated costs, value-based health care creates a total package price for reimbursement in which costs are risk adjusted according to the severity of the illness and associated comorbidities, but it does not separate payments for individual physicians or treatment centers. Such a cost model could create opportunities for significant cost reduction by lowering the total costs involved in care by eliminating redundant services, optimizing capacity, shortening cycle times, and measuring true costs associated with resource use.

Alternative methods of achieving total package pricing, such as not reimbursing physicians or facilities for preventable complications, have been proposed.[24] Many physicians choose to stay neutral on the topic of reimbursement for preventable complications. This attitude may be reducing the number of valid findings available to determine the advantages or disadvantages of this model.[16,24] Historically, delivery of health care services has been found to decline when providers are asked to contain costs.[25] The creation and wide implementation of care-cycle pricing as defined by Porter may create the same issues.

When current health care costs are examined within the context of Porter's hierarchical outcome model, it is apparent that outcome measurement focuses on tier 1 (ie, survival and health status achieved). As expensive new treatments and technology are introduced, health care costs increase but with potentially no improvement in survival. However, within the context of the 3-tiered outcome model, which provides broader measurement of outcomes, new treatments may result in opportunities for overall cost reduction; for example, by decreasing the time for a patient to return to work.[13] Opportunities for improvements in the process of recovery (tier 2) and health sustainability (tier 3) are also likely to lower costs.

APPLICATION OF VALUE-BASED HEALTH CARE

At the national level, Sweden and Denmark have shown the feasibility and impact of establishing national quality health care registries.[26] In the United States, universal outcome measurement systems and reporting have been mandated for programs in organ transplantation,[27] in vitro fertilization,[28] coronary care,[29] and dialysis care.[13] These programs have shown that outcome measurement is practical, is economically feasible, can provide acceptable risk adjustment, and can reduce variations in care across providers over time.[13] Value-based approaches have also been evaluated for diagnostic imaging services[30] and in pharmacologic settings to initiate value-based drug pricing for new cancer drugs.[31,32] The evaluation of value-based drug pricing in this setting indicated that it may be a more feasible option than government-mandated pricing of treatment drugs.[31] It is still too early to determine whether value-based pricing will work for diagnostic imaging services.[30]

In the early 2000s, The University of Texas MD Anderson Cancer Center implemented several of Porter's principles to create a more value-centered approach to cancer care. Cancer-specific medical outpatient practice units that comprised multiple disciplines were designed to address the full spectrum of care for a variety of malignancies.[33] For example, the Melanoma and Skin Center combines the expertise of medical oncologists, radiation oncologists, pathologists, surgical oncologists, radiologists, nurses, and physician's assistants with specialized training related to melanoma and skin-related cancers within a specific geographic location at the institution. Patients are scheduled to visit 1 clinic for their primary medical evaluation, where their diagnosis, treatment planning, and follow-up are located, allowing patients to be more connected with their care team. The overall transition to medical practice units has been successful at MD Anderson Cancer Center, although the 5-year process of transition was costly because it required additional hiring of support staff and a reorganization of many facilities. The documented outcomes have included increased patient satisfaction and the improved ability of physicians to treat a higher volume of patients in a more patient-centered manner.

The transition to outpatient medical practice units has been successful at MD Anderson largely because of the commitment of the faculty, who thought that patient care would benefit by their greater interaction with disease-specific specialists and that the reorganization would facilitate high-quality, high-volume care. One of the key aspects of the medical practice units at MD Anderson is that individual cases of complicated malignancies are presented and discussed in multidisciplinary planning conferences. After a review of a case history and relevant laboratory results, a multidisciplinary team of pathologists, radiologists, medical oncologists, surgical oncologists, and radiation oncologists determines an individualized treatment plan. In addition, these conferences are excellent teaching venues for staff and trainees. Other institutions, including the Roswell Park Cancer Institute, have also adopted this system of care by establishing multidisciplinary clinical teams to assess treatment options and to determine cost estimates for patients and insurance companies.[34]

One of the challenges of adopting the concept of IPUs has been determining the appropriate estimates of cost in light of the significant variation in treatment options for various malignancies. A pilot study was begun at the Roswell Park Cancer Institute in which Porter's care-cycle pricing was used for patients with early-stage breast cancer. However, the program was terminated because of operational issues and the inability of the cost care cycle to fully account for possible complications.[34]

Both MD Anderson and the Roswell Park Cancer Institute have shown successful outcomes when clinical specialties are combined to form multidisciplinary care teams. However, the challenges noted at Roswell Park with their pilot program revealed gaps in knowledge about disease-specific care cycles that must be addressed before value-based health care can be fully adopted.

DISCUSSION

The goal of outcome measurement is to inform and stimulate the improvement of health care practice. Evaluation of outcomes in a value-based health care system requires that competition for services be created from results and value, not reputation and facility.[17] This type of competition mimics other industries centered around market-based solutions.[35] Value-based health care creates competition around value, which is defined as benefit per dollar spent.[35]

According to Porter,[13] improving value in health care requires defining and measuring the total set of outcomes for a medical condition and determining the major risk factors associated with these outcomes. The proposed benefits of value-based health care include the potential for higher patient volume, more leverage in purchasing, and greater innovation and advances in medicine.[22] Furthermore, value-based health care could increase quality, efficiency, and overall patient satisfaction.[36] The higher volume of patients reduces cost and allows diffusion of cost among a larger population. In addition, the premise of identifying care-cycle costs allows patients and reimbursement agencies to have firm estimates for the cycle of care. According to the premises of Porter's model, physicians are able to treat patients with similar conditions with increased specialization and collaboration with other specialists, thereby creating more efficient health care as well as the potential for more rapid advances in research.[20]

There has been significant discussion and some criticism of Porter's model of value-based health care. Tilburt and colleagues[37] noted that such a model is payer centered rather than patient centered and that such a value equation would "reward mediocre outcomes delivered cheaply."[37] Others have argued that the adoption of the proposed value-based system may result in the elimination of components or amenities of treatment that have little impact on a disease but are meaningful to patients and care givers (eg, chaplain services, treatment room atmosphere, and development of patient-provider relationships).[37] Furthermore, critics argue that the disease-specific hierarchy does not account for patient satisfaction, family participation, or ability to return to work.[38] To achieve a truly value-based health care system, care-cycle pricing would be required for every disease and combination of diseases at multiple stages. Models such as those introduced by Porter are unlikely to be adequate for comorbidities, which can significantly complicate treatment pathways.[33] Furthermore, although in this system some cost diffusion among low-risk patients may be beneficial, too much diffusion may create an environment in which patients who do not have complications become overburdened by the costs of more complicated cases.

By shifting to a value-based method, the potential exists to create an industry in which services are based on predetermined pathways alone and clinical innovation and judgment are eliminated.[36] In addition, the cycle-of-care cost analysis may limit medical care to predetermined pathways. For example, in Porter's value-based health care model, treatments offered in clinical trials are not addressed and such a system may reduce the opportunities for patients to receive cutting-edge treatment. Although Porter is critical of patients choosing care based on the reputation of the facility or physician, some patients choose to travel to certain facilities because of the expanded opportunities for treatments that may not be available elsewhere.

An alternative to the value-based model has been proposed in which insurance programs are designed to reduce patient barriers to health care. Proponents of the value-based system argue that amenities, such as chaplain services, hospital atmosphere, and room amenities, could be offered as a selection of services that would be added to the base care-cycle cost.[39] Instead of using 1-size-fits-all modeling for health care costs, patients in the more customized value-based health care model who are deemed at clinically significant risk for complications or are expected to need more complicated treatments would be identified and treated according to different clinical pathways, such as more frequent screening, follow-up, or evaluations for complications.[40]

SUMMARY

Many opportunities exist for improving the current system of health care delivery. Despite the ongoing debate on how to reform the system, it is clear that some type of value-based system is needed to account for both quality and cost. To do so, it is imperative that health care providers define meaningful outcome metrics for specific medical conditions related to value. Comprehensive outcome measurement could encompass the full cycle of care, include multiple dimensions of care, and be conducted continuously for every patient. Several of Porter's tenets have been successfully implemented in cancer care, oral surgery, skin disease, and cardiologic care.[33,41–43] However, the widespread implementation of this system would likely require a significant increase in short-term costs. Because many facilities are currently facing critical budget shortfalls, even a short-term increase in costs may cripple the health care industry. Value-based health care offers the opportunity for new collaborations among multidisciplinary physicians but may also limit the ability to provide individualized patient care.

REFERENCES

1. Oliver A, Greenberg CC. Measuring outcomes in oncology treatment: the importance of patient-centered outcomes. Surg Clin North Am 2009;89(1):17–25, vii.
2. Donabedian A. The quality of care. How can it be assessed? JAMA 1988;260(12):1743–8.
3. Goldstein H, Spiegelhalter DJ. League tables and their limitations: statistical issues in comparison of institutional performance. J R Stat Soc 1996;159(3):385–443.
4. Grunfeld E, Urquhart R, Mykhalovskiy E, et al. Toward population-based indicators of quality end-of-life care: testing stakeholder agreement. Cancer 2008;112(10):2301–8.
5. Haydar Z, Gunderson J, Ballard DJ, et al. Accelerating best care in Pennsylvania: adapting a large academic system's quality improvement process to rural community hospitals. Am J Med Qual 2008;23(4):252–8.
6. Birkmeyer JD, Dimick JB, Birkmeyer NJ. Measuring the quality of surgical care: structure, process, or outcomes? J Am Coll Surg 2004;198(4):626–32.
7. Birkmeyer JD, Siewers AE, Finlayson EV, et al. Hospital volume and surgical mortality in the United States. N Engl J Med 2002;346(15):1128–37.
8. Hewitt M, Petitti D. Interpreting the volume-outcome relationship in the context of health care quality. Washington, DC: National Academy Press; 2001.
9. Earle CC, Neville BA, Landrum MB, et al. Evaluating claims-based indicators of the intensity of end-of-life cancer care. Int J Qual Health Care 2005;17(6):505–9.
10. Henke RM, McGuire TG, Zaslavsky AM, et al. Clinician- and organization-level factors in the adoption of evidence-based care for depression in primary care. Health Care Manage Rev 2008;33(4):289–99.
11. Hepner KA, Rowe M, Rost K, et al. The effect of adherence to practice guidelines on depression outcomes. Ann Intern Med 2007;147(5):320–9.
12. Kiefe CI, Weissman NW, Allison JJ, et al. Identifying achievable benchmarks of care: concepts and methodology. Int J Qual Health Care 1998;10(5):443–7.
13. Porter ME. Measuring health outcomes: the outcome hierarchy. Supplementary appendix 2 to What is value in health care? N Engl J Med 2010;363:2477–81.
14. Porter ME. Value in health care. Supplementary appendix 1 to What is value in health care? N Engl J Med 2010;263:2477–81.
15. Institute of Medicine. Crossing the quality chasm: a new health system for the 21st century. Washington, DC: National Academy Press; 2001.
16. Porter ME. A strategy for health care reform–toward a value-based system. N Engl J Med 2009;361(2):109–12.
17. Porter ME. Value-based health care delivery. Ann Surg 2008;248(4):503–9.
18. Committee on Redesigning Health Insurance Performance Measures, Payment, and Performance Improvement Programs. Performance measurement: accelerating improvement. Washington, DC: National Academy Press; 2006.
19. Porter ME. What is value in health care? N Engl J Med 2010;363(26):2477–81.
20. Feeley TW, Fly HS, Albright H, et al. A method for defining value in healthcare using cancer care as a model. J Healthc Manag 2010;55(6):399–411 [discussion: 411–2].
21. Teperi J, Porter ME, Vuorenkoski L, et al. The Finnish health care system: a value-based perspective. Helsinki (Finland): Sitra; 2009.

22. Porter ME, Teisberg EO. Redefining health care: creating value-based competition on results. Boston: Harvard Business School Press; 2006.
23. Strite S, Stuart ME. What is an evidence-based, value-based health care system? (part 1). Physician Exec 2005;31(1):50–4.
24. Hoff T, Soerensen C. No payment for preventable complications: reviewing the early literature for content, guidance, and impressions. Qual Manag Health Care 2011;20(1):62–75.
25. Steele JR, Reilly JD. Bundled payments: bundled risk or bundled reward? J Am Coll Radiol 2010;7(1):43–9.
26. Porter ME, Molander R. Outcomes measurement: learning from international experiences. Harvard University Working Paper 2010. Available at: http://www.hbs.edu/rhc/prior.html.2010. Accessed July 28, 2011.
27. Porter ME, Baron JF, Chacko JM, et al. The UCLA medical center: kidney transplantation. Boston: Harvard Business School; 2010. product no. 711410-PDF-ENG.
28. Porter ME, Rahim S, Tsai B. In-vitro fertilization: outcomes measurement. Boston: Harvard Business School; 2008. product no. 709403-PDF-ENG.
29. Auerbach AD, Hilton JF, Maselli J, et al. Case volume, quality of care, and care efficiency in coronary artery bypass surgery. Arch Intern Med 2010;170(14):1202–8.
30. Garrison LP Jr, Bresnahan BW, Higashi MK, et al. Innovation in diagnostic imaging services assessing the potential for value-based reimbursement. Acad Radiol 2011;18(9):1109–14.
31. Dranitsaris G, Ortega A, Lubbe MS, et al. A pharmacoeconomic modeling approach to estimate a value-based price for new oncology drugs in Europe. J Oncol Pharm Pract 2012;18(1):57–67.
32. Dranitsaris G, Truter I, Lubbe MS, et al. The application of pharmacoeconomic modelling to estimate a value-based price for new cancer drugs. J Eval Clin Pract 2012;18(2):343–51.
33. Pollock RE. Value-based health care: the MD Anderson experience. Ann Surg 2008;248(4):510–6 [discussion: 517–8].
34. Germain P. Barriers to the optimal rehabilitation of surgical cancer patients in the managed care environment: an administrator's perspective. J Surg Oncol 2007;95(5):386–92.
35. Porter ME, Teisberg EO. How physicians can change the future of health care. JAMA 2007;297(10):1103–11.
36. Rowe JW. Pay-for-performance and accountability: related themes in improving health care. Ann Intern Med 2006;145(9):695–9.
37. Tilburt JC, Montori VM, Shah ND. What is value in health care? N Engl J Med 2011;364(13):e26 [author reply: e26].
38. Cohen AJ. What is value in health care? N Engl J Med 2010;364(13):e26 [author reply: e26].
39. Shannon D. Managing the critical transition from volume to value. Physician Exec 2011;37(3):4–9.
40. Saini SD, Fendrick AM. Value-based insurance design: implications for gastroenterology. Clin Gastroenterol Hepatol 2010;8(9):767–9.
41. Abbott MM, Meara JG. Value-based cleft lip-cleft palate care: a progress report. Plast Reconstr Surg 2010;126(3):1020–5.
42. Freeman K, Marum M, Bottomley JM, et al. A psoriasis-specific model to support decision making in practice - UK experience. Curr Med Res Opin 2011;27(1):205–23.
43. Marciniak TA, Ellerbeck EF, Radford MJ, et al. Improving the quality of care for Medicare patients with acute myocardial infarction: results from the Cooperative Cardiovascular Project. JAMA 1998;279(17):1351–7.

Index

Note: Page numbers of article titles are in **boldface** type.

A

Adjuvant therapy, predicting benefit of adjuvant chemotherapy in colon cancer, 443
American College of Surgeons, National Surgical Quality Improvement Program, 371–373
American Society of Clinical Oncology, cancer care quality measure from, 369
    Quality Oncology Practice Initiative, 370–371
Appropriateness method, for use of surgical procedures in cancer patients, **479–486**
      appropriateness criteria for, 481–483
      implementation of appropriateness criteria, 483–484
Artificial neural networks, as prediction tool in surgical oncology, 440–441

B

Breast cancer, randomized controlled trials in, 450–455
      impact on practice, 450–454
      limitations of, 454–455

C

Cancer care, defining quality of, 368–369
    outcomes of. *See* Outcomes research.
Cancer Program Practice Profile Reports, from Commission on Cancer, 371
Cancer surgery. *See* Surgery.
Center for Translational Cancer Research, 494–495
Chemotherapy, adjuvant, predicting benefit in colon cancer, 443
Clinical trials. *See* Randomized controlled trials.
Colon cancer, lymph node staging standards in, 408–409
    predicting benefit of adjuvant chemotherapy in, 443
Commission on Cancer, National Cancer Data Base, **377–388**
    program for cancer care quality standards, 371
Community cancer centers, collaboration with, **487–495**
      Center for Translational Cancer Research, 494–495
      establishing multidisciplinary disease site centers, 492–494
      genetic counseling and gene testing, 490–491
      in Delaware, 489–490
      NCI Community Clinical Oncology Program (CCOP), 491–492
      participation in NCI's Community Cancer Centers Program (NCCCP), 488–489
Community Cancer Centers Program (NCCCP), 488–489
Community Clinical Oncology Program (CCOP), 491–492
Complications, postoperative, understanding mortality after high-risk cancer surgery, **389–395**
Cost issues, value-based health care, **497–506**

Surg Oncol Clin N Am 21 (2012) 507–513
doi:10.1016/S1055-3207(12)00040-3
1055-3207/12/$ – see front matter © 2012 Elsevier Inc. All rights reserved.
surgonc.theclinics.com

D

Delaware, state cancer control program in, 489–490
Disparities, racial, in cancer care and outcomes, **417–437**

E

Esophageal cancer, lymph node staging standards in, 412–413

F

Failure to rescue, understanding mortality after high-risk cancer surgery, 391–393

G

Gastric cancer, lymph node staging standards in, 412
Gastrointestinal (GI) cancer, lymph node staging standards in, **407–416**
    history of, 408
    in colon cancer, 408–409
    in esophageal cancer, 412–413
    in gastric cancer, 412
    in pancreatic cancer, 410–411
    in rectal cancer, 409–410
Genetic counseling, collaborative approach with community cancer centers, 490–491
Genetic testing, collaborative approach with community cancer centers, 490–491

H

Health care, value-based. See Value-based health care/
Hospitals, rates of unexpected readmissions after major cancer surgery, **397–405**
Human factor analysis, of patient safety in surgical oncology, **467–478**
    case study, 474
    in the OR, 470–473
    methodologies, 469–470
    theoretical models, 468–469

I

Integrated practice units, in value-based health care, 500–501

L

Lymph nodes, staging standards in GI cancer, **407–416**
    history of, 408
    in colon cancer, 408–409
    in esophageal cancer, 412–413
    in gastric cancer, 412
    in pancreatic cancer, 410–411
    in rectal cancer, 409–410
Lymphadenectomy, lymph node staging standards in GI cancer, **407–416**

M

Monitoring, of delivery of cancer care, with National Cancer Data Base, **377–388**
Mortality, variation in, after high-risk cancer surgery, **389–395**
    failure to rescue, 391–393
    future directions, 393–394
    reasons for, 390
    recent advances in knowledge, 390–391
Multidisciplinary disease site centers, in community cancer centers, 492–494

N

National Cancer Data Base, for monitoring delivery of cancer care, **377–388**
    enhanced data systems of, 379–386
        evidence-based cancer care quality measures, 380–382
        increasing coverage, quality, and timeliness of data, 384–385
        linkage to other data sources and special studies, 383–384
        quality benchmarks and performance data, 384
        standardization of reporting, 382–383
        training of health service researchers, 385–386
    structure and organization, 378–379
National Cancer Institute (NCI), Community Cancer Centers Program (NCCCP), 488–489
    Community Clinical Oncology Program (CCOP), 491–492
National Quality Foundation, cancer care quality measure from, 369
National Surgical Quality Improvement Program, from American College of Surgeons, 371–373
Neural networks, artificial, as prediction tool in surgical oncology, 440–441
Nomograms, as prediction tool in surgical oncology, 440–441
    for predicting recurrence after radical prostatectomy, 442–443
    in thyroid nodules, 441–442

O

Oncology, surgical, outcomes research in. *See* Outcomes research.
Operating room (OR), human factor analysis of surgical oncology patient safety in, **467–478**
    case study, 474
    in the OR, 470–473
    methodologies, 469–470
    theoretical models, 468–469
Outcome hierarchy, in value-based health care, 499–500
Outcomes research, in surgical oncology, 367–506
    appropriate use of surgical procedures in cancer patient, **479–486**
        appropriateness criteria for cancer patients, 481–483
        appropriateness method, 481
        implementation of appropriateness criteria, 483–484
    collaboration with community cancer centers, **487–495**
        Center for Translational Cancer Research, 494–495
        establishing multidisciplinary disease site centers, 492–494
        genetic counseling and gene testing, 490–491
        in Delaware, 489–490

Outcomes (*continued*)
        NCI Community Clinical Oncology Program (CCOP), 491–492
        participation in NCI's Community Cancer Centers Program, 488–489
      lymph node staging standards in GI cancer, **407–416**
        history of, 408
        in colon cancer, 408–409
        in esophageal cancer, 412–413
        in gastric cancer, 412
        in pancreatic cancer, 410–411
        in rectal cancer, 409–410
      monitoring delivery of cancer care, **377–388**
        future work on, 386
        National Cancer Data Base, 378–386
      patient safety, human factor analysis of, **467–478**
        case study, 474
        in the OR, 470–473
        methodologies, 469–470
        theoretical models, 468–469
      prediction tools, **439–447**
        artificial neural networks, prediction tables, and nomograms, 440–441
        evaluating and comparing, 443–444
        examples of, 441–443
        future of, 444–445
      quality improvement initiatives, **367–375**
        currently available measures, 369–370
        defining quality cancer care, 368–369
        future directions, 373
        programs measuring cancer care quality, 370–373
      racial differences and disparities in care and outcomes, **417–437**
        health care policy implications, 428–430
        mechanisms underlying, 418–426
        research recommendations and future directions, 426–428
        scope of problem, 417–418
      randomized controlled trials in, **449–466**
        additional lessons from, 459–460
        future directions encompassing lessons learned from, 460–461
        in breast cancer, 450–455
        in rectal cancer, 455–459
        relevance in surgery, 450
      unexpected readmissions after major cancer surgery, **397–405**
      value-based health care, **497–506**
        application of, 502–503
        costs of care, 501–502
        integrated practice units, 500–501
        outcomes hierarchy, 499–500
      variations in mortality after high-risk cancer surgery, **389–395**
        failure to rescue, 391–393
        future directions, 393–394
        reasons for, 390
        recent advances in knowledge, 390–391
Overuse, appropriate use of surgical procedures in cancer patients, **479–486**

P

Pancreatic cancer, lymph node staging standards in, 410–411
Patient safety. *See* Safety, patient.
Postoperative complications, understanding mortality after high-risk cancer surgery,
    389–395
Prediction tools, in surgical oncology, **439–447**
    artificial neural networks, prediction tables, and nomograms, 440–441
    evaluating and comparing, 443–444
    examples of, 441–443
        for benefit of adjuvant chemotherapy in colon cancer, 443
        for disease recurrence after radical prostatectomy, 442–443
        for malignancy in thyroid nodules, 441–442
        for pathologic stage in prostate cancer, 441
    future of, 444–445
Prostate cancer, nomograms predicting recurrence after radical prostatectomy, 442
    predicting pathologic stage in, 441

Q

Quality improvement initiatives. *See also* Outcomes research.
    in surgical oncology, **367–375**
        currently available measures, 369–370
            American Society of Clinical Oncology, 369
            gaps in, 370
            National Quality Forum, 369
            other, 369–370
        defining quality cancer care, 368–369
        future directions, 373
        programs measuring cancer care quality, 370–373
            American Society of Clinical Oncology, 370–371
            Commission on Cancer, 371
            National Surgical Quality Improvement Program, 371–373
Quality Oncology Practice Initiative, 370–371

R

Racial differences, and disparities in cancer care and outcomes, **417–437**
        health care policy implications, 428–430
            expand use of active comanagement, 430
            expand use of patient navigators, 429
            improve access to care, 428–429
            increase adherence to best practices, 430
            increase diversity in physician workforce, 429
        mechanisms underlying, 418–426
            cancer stage, 418
            failure to provide optimal treatment, 421–426
            treatment toxicity and efficacy, 419–421
            tumor biology, 418–419
        research recommendations and future directions, 426–428
            consider alternative research methodologies, 427–428

Racial (*continued*)
      improve collection of sociodemographic data, 427
      use optimal risk adjustment methodology, 427
   scope of problem, 417–418
Randomized controlled trials, in surgical oncology, **449–466**
   additional lessons from, 459–460
   future directions encompassing lessons learned from, 460–461
   in breast cancer, 450–455
   in rectal cancer, 455–459
   relevance in surgery, 450
Rapid Quality Reporting System, from Commission on Cancer, 371, 384–385
Readmissions, unexpected, after major cancer surgery, **397–405**
Rectal cancer, lymph node staging standards in, 409–410
   randomized controlled trials in, 455–459
Registries, National Cancer Data Base, **377–388**
Rescue, failure to, and mortality after high-risk cancer surgery, 391–393
Research, on racial differences and disparities in cancer care, recommendations and future
   directions for, 426–428
   consider alternative research methodologies, 427–428
   improve collection of sociodemographic data, 427
   use optimal risk adjustment methodology, 427
  outcomes. *See* Outcomes research.

S

Safety, patient, human factor analysis of, in surgical oncology, **467–478**
   case study, 474
   in the OR, 470–473
   methodologies, 469–470
   theoretical models, 468–469
Staging, lymph node standards in GI cancer, **407–416**
   history of, 408
   in colon cancer, 408–409
   in esophageal cancer, 412–413
   in gastric cancer, 412
   in pancreatic cancer, 410–411
   in rectal cancer, 409–410
Surgery, appropriate use of surgical procedures in cancer patients, **479–486**
   outcomes research in oncology. *See* Outcomes research.
   randomized controlled trials in oncologic, **449–466**
   unexpected readmissions after major cancer, **397–405**
   variation in mortality after high-risk cancer, **389–395**

T

Thyroid nodules, nomogram predicting malignancy in, 441–442
Translational cancer research, 494–495
Trials. *See* Randomized controlled trials.

U

Underuse, appropriate use of surgical procedures in cancer patients, **479–486**

V

Value-based health care, surgical oncologist's perspective on, **497–506**
    application of, 502–503
    costs of care, 501–502
    integrated practice units, 500–501
    outcomes hierarchy, 499–500

Moving?

Make sure your subscription moves with you!

To notify us of your new address, find your **Clinics Account Number** (located on your mailing label above your name), and contact customer service at:

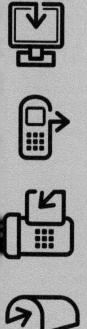

Email: journalscustomerservice-usa@elsevier.com

800-654-2452 (subscribers in the U.S. & Canada)
314-447-8871 (subscribers outside of the U.S. & Canada)

Fax number: 314-447-8029

Elsevier Health Sciences Division
Subscription Customer Service
3251 Riverport Lane
Maryland Heights, MO 63043

*To ensure uninterrupted delivery of your subscription, please notify us at least 4 weeks in advance of move.

Printed and bound by CPI Group (UK) Ltd, Croydon, CR0 4YY

03/10/2024

01040442-0013